THE VETERINARY RECEPTIONIST
Essential Skills for Client Care

D1073542

To all those people that are NOT 'just' a receptionist!

For Elsevier:

Commissioning Editor: Rita Demetriou-Swanwick
Development Editor: Louisa Welch
Project Manager: Kerrie-Anne Jarvis
Designer: George Ajayi
Illustration Manager: Merlyn Harvey
Illustrator: Graeme Chambers, David Banks, Cactus

THE VETERINARY RECEPTIONIST

Essential Skills for Client Care

SECOND EDITION

John R. Corsan NCA, NDA
Principal, Vetlink Ltd, UK

Adrian R. Mackay BSc(Hons), DipM, MCIM, MBA
Managing Partner, Duncan Alexander & Wilmshurst, UK

Edinburgh London New York Oxford Philadelphia St Louis Sydney Toronto 2008

SAUNDERS
ELSEVIER

First published 2001
Second edition 2008

ISBN: 978-0-7020-2928-8

British Library Cataloguing in Publication Data
A catalogue record for this book is available from the British Library

Library of Congress Cataloging in Publication Data
A catalog record for this book is available from the Library of Congress

Working together to grow
libraries in developing countries

www.elsevier.com | www.bookaid.org | www.sabre.org

 ELSEVIER   BOOK AID International   Sabre Foundation

ELSEVIER   your source for books, journals and multimedia in the health sciences

www.elsevierhealth.com

The Publisher's policy is to use paper manufactured from sustainable forests

Printed in China

Contents

Foreword   vii

The Perfect Receptionist   ix

CHAPTER 1   CLIENT SERVICE DEFINED   1

CHAPTER 2   MAKE YOUR FIRST IMPRESSIONS COUNT   26

CHAPTER 3   FOCUS ON YOUR CLIENT   32

CHAPTER 4   MAKING THE CLIENT FEEL 'SPECIAL'   42

CHAPTER 5   TELEPHONE SKILLS   58

CHAPTER 6   PROFESSIONAL UNDER PRESSURE   70

CHAPTER 7   PROFIT FROM COMPLAINTS   98

CHAPTER 8   CLIENT SERVICE SOLUTIONS   119

CHAPTER 9   FUNDAMENTALS OF FIRST AID   136

CHAPTER 10   LABELLING AND DISPENSING   144

Appendix Action Plan   156

Index   157

Foreword

Veterinary practice has come a long way over the past 20 years and the pet owner should be able to choose a veterinary practice with confidence, knowing that their pet will receive the best of care. New medicines, not just antibiotic, but therapy for a range of ailments, are now available. New surgical techniques, developed in centres of excellence, are being used in general practice. Young veterinary graduates are qualifying with a vast range of knowledge that, in the right circumstances, will be nurtured and brought to benefit the animals under their care.

Another development is the role of support staff within the practice. Obviously veterinary nurses have made an enormous contribution to efficient clinical care and many practices now demand that the ratio of veterinary surgeons to veterinary nurses is 1:1, such is their assistance in ensuring excellent patient care. Practice managers, once an aspiration of many practices, are now considered to be absolutely essential to sort out the plethora of paperwork, HR resource issues and the all-present health and safety regulations.

As this book reminds the reader, the veterinary profession is a service industry and increasingly the profession must recognise that veterinary surgeons exist not just to look after the needs of animals – their health, welfare and illnesses – but must also service the needs of their owners – the clients. It is recognised that clients now have higher expectations of their practice and sadly, are correspondingly more likely to sue if the service falls short of expectations.

At the forefront of this contact with the client is the veterinary receptionist. The 'Perfect Receptionist' may occasionally be found but not everyone has the charisma necessary to instantly achieve the art of client service: that is, the ability to make people feel special. This book has in-depth advice on how to achieve perfection in this art but also has chapters devoted to ensuring that the veterinary receptionist has an excellent understanding of the work of the veterinary surgeons and nurses in the practice.

The chapter on labelling and dispensing medicines is particularly relevant at a time when the Veterinary Medicines Directorate (VMD) has shaken up the old Medicines Act from 1968 and produced new Regulations, which are updated and in some cases, quite substantially altered, on an annual basis. Particularly relevant to the veterinary receptionist is the section on 'Supply when a veterinary surgeon is not present'. It is exactly this sort of professionalism that practices must adhere to because the VMD have given fair warning that veterinary surgeons must be accountable for their actions and must keep within the letter of the law.

There are so many books dedicated to the needs of veterinary nurses but few for ancillary staff so this volume is very welcome. Experienced reception staff will find much 'further education' in its pages and beginners will benefit from a considerable resource of practical knowledge delivered by the authors in a clear, concise way with lovely touches of humour to keep the reader stimulated. Veterinary surgeons and nurses will also benefit from dipping into this book and the authors are to be commended for their work.

Freda Scott-Park (Dr)
BVM&S, PhD Hon.DVM&S, MRCVS

The Perfect Receptionist

Sandie Agar VN

The Perfect Receptionist is resolutely cheerful in the face of all adversity (even the Principal in a bad mood).

She always wears a welcoming smile and has eye contact with each and every member of the waiting-room (for a maximum of 3 seconds).

She has the memory of an elephant, demonstrates unfailing tact, has the wisdom of Solomon and exercises tolerance and patience in all situations.

Being kind to all things furry and scaly, she does not drown parentally uncontrolled children in the fish tank, but is firm with them, gives them comics to read and politely requests that next time they remain at home.

Her sense of humour is always apparent but never inappropriate.

She comforts the bereaved and distressed, reassures the timid, soothes the nervous, calms the fractious and even changes the odd nappy on occasions.

She is always smartly dressed and retains her well-groomed appearance even after wrestling with rottweilers or rescuing trapped budgies from behind the consulting-room sink.

She maintains the waiting-room in spotless condition, torn comics are removed to the bin immediately, while puddles (and worse) are cleared away swiftly and efficiently.

Pictures always hang straight and posters are never torn or crumpled.

The area under the desk is tidy, all leaflets are constrained in alphabetical order in neat rows. The appointment/message book is carefully aligned on the desk top, a precise 3.75 cm from the edge and its corners are never allowed to curl.

She loves the computer, can type speedily and accurately and dusts the keyboard's crevices daily.

All enquiries are dealt with the day before they arrive. She is meticulous in her note-taking and passes on messages with unerring accuracy, checking afterwards that they have been received.

She is able to provide tea and biscuits (chocolate) on demand for the flagging vets, harassed nurses and clients in need.

She is able to charm money from the wallets with the skill of an Indian snake-charmer, never gives the wrong change and provides a receipt while answering the phone after precisely 3 rings, even when all lines are ringing in unison.

She works long hours for a mere pittance and is always willing to do extra.

This paragon of all virtues wears wings and a halo and thankfully does not exist – she would be so hard to live with.

Chapter 1

Client service defined

SO WHAT *IS* CLIENT SERVICE

CLIENT SERVICE – WHY BOTHER?

After all, clients have sick animals so they *need* to bring their animals to us… or at least get a vet to their herd, flock or bay gelding! Let's face it, we're pretty busy right now… don't they realize how much we've got to do before we close? Hmm…. That's probably not what you think (otherwise you would not have picked up this book!), but how many times have you been shopping lately and felt that the person serving you was thinking along those lines?

Most professionals and most professional firms appreciate the importance of client service – that is, serving the needs of clients. High street banks, law firms, fast-food restaurants, travel agencies, hairdressers, hospitals, your local (private!) dentist, and so on, are examples of organizations that exist only to provide services to their customers or clients.

Your veterinary practice is also a professional service firm, but does your practice provide such excellent service that your clients will never look elsewhere?

Reported in the earlier edition of this book, the authors were involved in a MORI poll of 1000 dog and 1000 cat owners that aimed to understand their attitudes to veterinary services. There were some interesting findings. One of the first things that they were asked was how satisfied were they about the overall service levels provided by their usual veterinary practice. To measure the differences in response, a five-point scale ranging from 1 for very unhappy through to 5 for very happy was used. This developed a scale of 'chuffedness' (Figure 1.1). What do you think the average score was for all clients evaluating all the various elements of the things that affected how they felt about the services provided by their veterinary practice?

Four, maybe four and a half?

Sadly, while you may feel that that would be what your practice might score, you must remember that here we are asking all owners looking at all the various factors that affect their perception. Remember, too, that we were not just asking the regular visitors to veterinary practices. Included in the survey were all those people that only take their pet to the surgery for emergencies.

The average score countrywide then was only 3.2. In other words, the opinion of clients on average was pretty non-committal; they tended not to have a

1

1	2	3	4	5
☹		☺		☺
Very unhappy	Unhappy	Neither happy nor unhappy	Happy	Very happy

Figure 1.1   A 'Chuffed Chart' to gauge client opinion on service satisfaction

particularly positive view or a particularly negative view. Sure, there were people who had a much more positive view, some scoring five on the scale. These people one could imagine doing cartwheels across the car park once they had finished paying – so happy are they with your service that they just can't wait to come back in and spend some more. Others, of course, at the other end of the scale are planning to sue you if they could because they did not like the colour of your floor tiles!

But should we worry that the score is only around three? Well, just reflect for a moment that your high street bank would have a mean score of around 4.1 on the same scale. And how do you feel about their charges?

An interesting finding from the MORI poll was discovered when the various groups were asked about their loyalty to their particular practice. Those people who scored their practice four out of five over all the various service issues were asked how loyal they were to their practice. In other words, if there were an alternative practice within easy reach of where they lived, that offered the same value for money as their current practice, would they switch?

What percentage do you think would move? Five percent? Maybe ten?

No. It was surprising to find that a staggering 20% – that is one in five clients – would move to another practice if the opportunity arose. And they are all above average on the chuffed-chart!

Now, we asked the people who scored their practice five out of five. This was a smaller group than the people who scored four but, nonetheless, a significant number of clients. One would think that these were pretty committed to their vet. Sadly not. Even among this group of what one might expect to call your practices' 'bonded clients' a surprising 5% – or one in twenty – would move on.

Now, hands up. Who wants a 5% pay cut next year? No? Well, of course not. What happens is that for every departing client the practice hopes to gain new ones. Unfortunately, it is estimated that it costs about six times as much to recruit a new client than it does to hold on to an existing client. Moreover, with the increasing growth of cat owners over dog owners, and more 'furries' like rabbits,

QUO VADIS – OR WHERE NOW?

The 'Quo vadis' study was conducted by Veterinary Business Development – owners of *The Veterinary Business Journal* and *Veterinary Times* – more recently and designed to look into the future of veterinary practice. Among the findings, they discovered that clients in the last five years prior to the study had become yet more demanding: higher expectations (of clinical success) – particularly in small animal and mixed practices – and higher service requirements across all types of clients. More worryingly, it appeared that companion clients would be more likely to sue!

The reasons given for pet owners moving from one practice to another was interesting. While one fifth changed because they simply moved house, 31% cited the practice as being too expensive, while 22% said that the practice was unfriendly or unhelpful. As we shall discover, both these last two issues can be addressed by the practice: both veterinary and support staff. On the other hand, cattle, sheep and pig farmers seemed to be more loyal to their practices with around 90% of each client type saying that they were 'not very... or not at all...' likely to change.

Practices were asked how they might compete with the growing competition coming from veterinary clinics in pet superstores; they concluded that they would need to offer 'better service' (51%) or a more 'personal service' (32%). Indeed, in general terms, practices were aware that in order to increase their business and stave off the competition, they would need to 'increase the awareness and educate their clients (about their facilities and manage their expectations)' (51%) and 'improve service aspects' (30%).

where these owners usually spend less, every practice needs to hold onto its client-base and ensure that it can move its clients up the chuffed-chart!

Clients cannot realistically judge the level of clinical care you give (although they consider themselves experts having just 'looked it up on the web'), but they can and do judge the level of service they receive. Naturally, they will have an opinion about the clinical side of your care and any doubts they have about the quality of the veterinary medicine are usually resolved by clarifying the client's misunderstanding. But service levels are different. In the client's eyes, the only major factor that distinguishes you and makes you unique from other practices is the service you provide. Therefore, striving for excellence in client service is essential. And, if service differentiates one practice from the other, who delivers that service? The people, of course. People like you and all your colleagues in the practice.

Now, while the reasons for clients moving from one practice to another are many and varied, the majority of the causes of dissatisfaction have much to do with the relationship the client has with the veterinary surgeon – and how he or she relates to them. While you might like to get all the veterinary surgeons to study this book, we have to recognize that working in the 'front line' at reception can also have a significant impact on clients.

As we shall see in the chapter on handling complaints (Chapter 7), client recommendations are very powerful; satisfied clients will recommend you to four or five other people, whereas dissatisfied clients could tell upwards of ten people about their experiences. Studies have shown that for every dissatisfied client who does complain, more than 20 say nothing – they just don't return. Measuring client satisfaction in your practice can help prevent these losses and maintain a more stable, satisfied client base.

But why bother? You may feel that exceptional client care only benefits the partners – they are the ones with a financial stake in the business. But what is the purpose of veterinary practice? It is not just a money-making machine. The purpose of your veterinary practice has much to do with animal health and welfare, healing sick animals and maintaining the health of the well. And the curious thing you may have noticed about animals – be they farm animals or pets – is that they don't call the vet themselves or make their own way to the practice and they don't carry cash, cheque books or credit cards. (Mind you, you probably know a few clients that don't seem to carry any either!) So, in order to do the best for the animal kingdom, like it or not, the practice must take care of the human dimension before it can even start to affect animal care.

Remember, there are three parties in the client care equation, illustrated in Figure 1.2. Let us consider for a moment the bonds between the three parties. That between the pet and the client (A) is very strong – they become 'the babies', part of the family. The practice wants the client-to-practice bond (B) to be strong, too, as this encourages loyalty – and some clients will say that they must see *their* vet and become very protective about the relationship. But what of the pet-to-practice bond (C)? This is one area that people at reception particularly can influence and we will return to this in Chapter 4 on how to make the client feel special.

Box 1.1 summarizes a 10-point guide to 'What is a client?' It highlights the importance of the client to the practice – that without clients (and their animals) there is no practice.

So, we know it is important, but let us answer the question, what is client service?

Box 1.1   What is a client? Adapted from IBM client charter – why not publish this list in the staff rest area?

'A client is the most important person *ever* in this practice… in person, on the telephone, or even by e-mail.'

'A client is a crucial part of this practice… he or she is the lifeblood of this practice.'

'A client is not dependent on us… we are dependent on him/her.'

'A client is not an interruption to our work…he or she is the purpose of it.'

'A client is doing us a favour by giving us the opportunity to serve them –we are not doing them a favour by serving them.'

'A client is not someone to argue or match wits with… *nobody ever won an argument with a client!*'

'A client is not a cold statistic – they are flesh and blood humans with feelings and emotions like our own.'

'A client is a person who brings us his/her needs, wants and desires. It is our job to handle them profitably both to him/her and to ourselves.'

'A client deserves the most courteous and attentive treatment we can give.'

'A client pays our wages!'

CLIENT SERVICE DEFINED

Simply put, client service is the ability to meet client requirements.

Unlike products that are solid, tangible entities, services are *experienced* and the veterinary surgeon's duty, as the primary service provider, is as much about managing the client's experience as in providing technical expertise. Box 1.2 is a useful list summarizing what clients might reasonably expect from their veterinary surgeon in order to create a strong bond between themselves and the practice (Bond 'B' in Figure 1.2).

However, for the veterinary receptionist there is a key role in managing the client-to-practice interface. Moreover, as the veterinary receptionist, you are the first point of contact in so many of the service situations experienced by clients as they deal with the practice for so many of the veterinary services and product sales offered.

One of the fundamentals of client service, established by David Maister in 1984 is his 'First Law of Service:

$$\text{SATISFACTION} = \text{PERCEPTION} - \text{EXPECTATION}$$

If the client perceives better than expected service then satisfaction is high; but if the service received did not meet expectations then satisfaction is low (Figure 1.3). The aim of all the members of a veterinary practice is that every client who visits the practice comes away very satisfied with the service they have received. That is the way business is built.

WHAT IS QUALITY CLIENT SERVICE?

Who is the best judge of the quality of the service you provide – the senior partner, the practice manager? No, of course not. The best judges of client service are the clients themselves. Unfortunately, every one is different and what one person might perceive as excellent service may be woefully inadequate for another!

Box 1.2   The 'top ten' things that clients want when bringing their pet to the surgery

To create a strong bond with the practice, clients want their veterinary surgeons to:
- Respect that their time is valuable too by being on time for their appointments
- Make them feel valued as individuals, rather than be treated as numbers
- Establish a personal contact or rapport of the appropriate kind with them
- Greet them and their pets by name
- Show interest in and enthusiasm for them, their pets (and even their children)
- Show affection for their pet
- Handle the pet kindly and not use unnecessary restraint
- Explain what they are doing in terms that they can understand without being patronizing
- Give an accurate estimate of the fees (and other expenses where possible)
- Take phone calls from them or call back promptly whenever possible

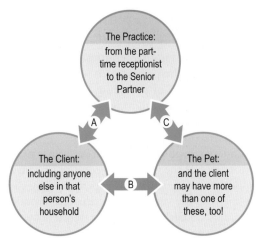

Figure 1.2 The three parties in the client care equation

Satisfaction can be extended to include a perception of quality. The highly satisfied client will feel they have received a high-quality service, whereas the dissatisfied client will be disappointed by the quality of service.

WHAT IS MEANT BY QUALITY?

Quality is whatever you and your clients want it to be.

Take the example of a high street fruit market. The greengrocer had a whole range of fruit on his stall displayed on the artificial grass-effect cloth. At one end he had a pile of shiny, red apples at 55 pence a kilo. At the other end he had a similar pile of equally shiny, red apples at 95 pence a kilo. When asked the difference

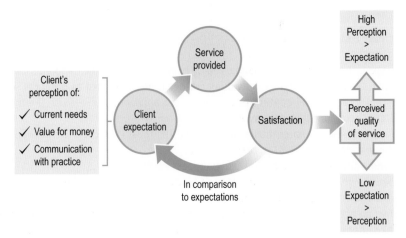

Figure 1.3 Factors influencing a client's perception of service quality

between the two, what do you think he said? Different apples, different freshness, different grade? No, none of these. He said that those at 95 pence a kilo were for those people who *wanted* to pay 95 pence a kilo! And if you think that is a little strange, Marks & Spencer have built a billion pound food hall business out of just that. You know the slogan: 'Good food costs less at Sainsburys ...' Well, good food costs slightly more at Marks & Spencer. And what about Fortnum & Masons? Do you think a one pound/454 g jar of marmalade at £9.99 is good value? Well, don't worry; you are in the majority who perhaps doesn't think so. But there are enough people, it would appear, who do think it does represent good value – or otherwise Fortnum's would not be able to charge those prices!

It all depends on what your clients perceive to be quality.

Some clients are quite happy paying relatively high prices for vaccinations compared to neighbouring practices, others are happy with getting the lowest price.

Whatever the client's position on quality, there are some basic issues regarding quality that are worth recognizing within the reception environment.

Quality is:

> *Represented by intangibles* (things you can only see) such as the friendly smile, the tidy reception area, the polite voice over the phone. These are things that each individual in the reception can influence directly.
>
> *Related to the situation* where different situations require different standards of quality. However, 'high' or 'low' quality does not exist – either the service meets the client's requirements or it does not. Compare a 'Brewer's Fayre' or 'Beefeater' pub restaurant with a McDonalds; the pub restaurant does not have 'higher' quality than McDonalds, it is just that their customers have different needs. Diners in the pub restaurant want 'honest' food and service to match the occasion – a working lunch mid-week or a meal with the family at the weekend; McDonalds customers also want good value food, but more often than not in a hurry. (But remember even 'hurry' has different connotations for different people. While the majority does not like to wait or queue in a McDonalds, no one wants to be treated in an off-hand way. Hence, the realignment of their original promotional strategy to 'We've got time for you.')
>
> So, how will your approach to a given client differ when they arrive for an annual vaccination compared to a euthanasia appointment?
>
> *Dynamic and constantly requiring reassessment and change.* Quality can become dated as requirements change. Compare the needs of customers shopping for their weekly groceries in the village store in years past, where personal service and perhaps time to gossip may have been important, to the customer rushing to the modern supermarket, where range of goods and speed of checkout are valued today. However, again, there is a progression in service delivery at the superstore. New services like coffee shops, crèches, packing and carryout services, 24-hour opening, cash withdrawals, loyalty cards, and more.
>
> What is going to have to be changed in your practice in order that you can keep up with the ever changing (and increasing) demands of veterinary clients? The authors know of one practice in a commuter town to London that opens at 6.00 a.m. to book animals (mostly cats) in for their annual booster vaccination and health check. Clients can collect their pets up to

10.00 p.m. that evening. Yes, they do have the space to look after the cats all day and they do charge their clients accordingly.

Relative: what one person perceives as quality may not be as important to another. Some clients would really appreciate a phone call as soon as possible from the practice to confirm that their animal is OK after surgery, others are happy to call themselves after three o'clock, others to wait until they come in to collect their animal later that evening.

Attention to detail: a quality practice must show that quality everywhere at all times. It is not adequate simply to have longer appointments and charge higher fees – the practice must always be clean, the staff must always be friendly, all clients always get a call back from someone in the practice that same day, and so on.

HOW DO CLIENTS DEFINE QUALITY?

> I don't care how much you know until I know how much you care
> ...A client's plea!

The measurement of satisfaction/quality is still in an early stage because there is no standard formula that precisely matches all individual client requirements. In addition, quality is affected by many variables, from individual veterinary practice's interpretation of what clients want as service through to client compliance with instructions about animal care.

Research in the USA has produced a new and widely accepted set of 10 client quality evaluation criteria. They help to highlight the importance of identifying quality criteria issues that are actually important to clients and that clients really do use to evaluate the 'quality' of the service provided. These are often different from the criteria professionals such as veterinary surgeons think are important to clients, and which they might use to evaluate quality of what they provide.

1. *Reliability.* How consistent and dependable is the practice every time I interact?
2. *Access.* Is the vet easily accessible and service delivered with little waiting?
3. *Credibility.* Can the pet owner trust the practice – are they honest?
4. *Security.* Are the risks and dangers known and acceptable – cost of the procedure and well-being of the pet?
5. *Knowledge.* Does the practice make every effort to understand the needs of the client?
6. *Responsiveness.* How willing are employees to provide the services?
7. *Competence.* Do all staff have the knowledge and skills required to give good service?
8. *Courtesy.* Are all staff polite and considerate to clients?
9. *Communication.* Does the practice clearly explain its products and services in ways that I can understand?
10. *Tangibles.* Does the appearance of the personnel, the surgery and waiting areas and other tangible evidence of the service, project an image of high quality?

Perceived value = 30%

Perceived value = 70%

Vet advice

Service delivery

Cost = 70%

Cost = 30%

Figure 1.4   A client's judgement of the value received compared to the costs to the practice of providing the advice of service delivery

Note here that price of the service does not appear in the list. This issue will be picked up in the section on page 13.

Chapter 2 has some further ways that client service is evaluated by clients and presents a series of key skills and behaviours recognized as being important to client care. They are presented as a self-appraisal questionnaire that is useful for your own interest and when shared with your colleagues, a way of moving together as a team. The team dynamics of client care is discussed later in this chapter.

In general terms, as Figure 1.4 aims to illustrate, while the cost to the practice of providing the professional advice is high, its impact on the client is less than the higher perceived value of the service delivered, which costs the practice less. For example, getting access to see their veterinary surgeon of choice or receiving a phone call back promptly is perceived to be of more value to the client than the most intricate and complex diagnosis!

'STEP-BY-STEP' SERVICE IN PRACTICE

If we look at many of the everyday activities in veterinary practice, we can see that clients progress 'step-by-step' in a process that starts with the client recognizing the need to seek veterinary advice, contacting the practice and finishes with the client leaving. Analysis of these steps helps identify where the receptionist has a role in influencing the quality of the service. It should be noted that there are many areas where the veterinary surgeon in particular or the practice in general has to make decisions about applying extra resources to improve the service delivery. The trick is to know the difference between what receptionists can do and what the practice must do to make a difference. (If, as the receptionist, you have any problems convincing partners or practice managers – just lend them your copy of this book!)

So how do we analyse these step-by-step service processes? The method is simple: identify a service and write, in step-wise fashion, what should happen ideally as the client goes through their thought processes and activities in receiving a given service. These are the basic steps in the client care process. Then, for every step, identify all the things that could go wrong. This is where the client could fall through the stairs and not continue on their journey through your client service process. By identifying all potential problems, you are in a position to control and prevent them before they happen. You are, thus, controlling the quality of service that you give. Step-by-Step service process analysis can become a practical way to apply quality control in your practice (Figures 1.5–1.7).

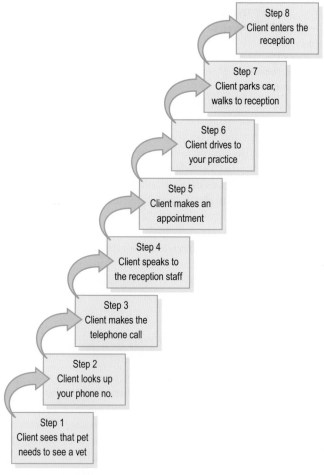

Figure 1.5   The Step-by-Step process for a client making an appointment and arriving at the practice

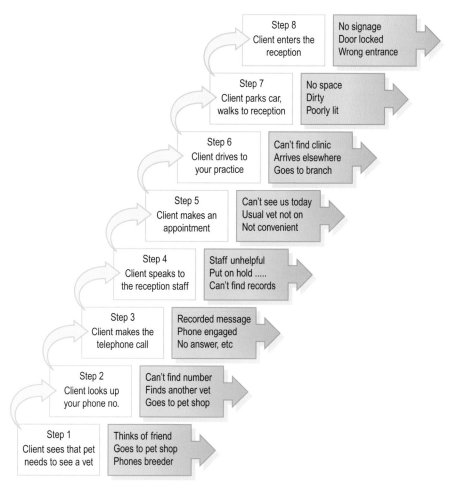

Figure 1.6   The possible reasons why the process of making an appointment and getting to the practice might go wrong for the client – why the client might slip through the steps!

Some suggestions to stop them falling through the gaps might be:

1. Make your practice a centre of excellence in animal health and welfare and *the* place to turn to for advice – not just for emergencies. All your publicity activities should be geared to putting the practice 'on the map' for all animal owners and a place where they feel they can drop in informally to pick-up information, leaflets and pet products (non-prescription, of course) without the formality of an appointment.
2. If you go into your local stationers and pick up a box of labels, say 24 to a sheet, you'll be able to print out hundreds of sticky labels with your practice name and phone number for pennies each. Why not send a couple with each of your vaccine reminder cards in an envelope – and clients can stick them on their Yellow Pages® cover or in their phone book, etc.

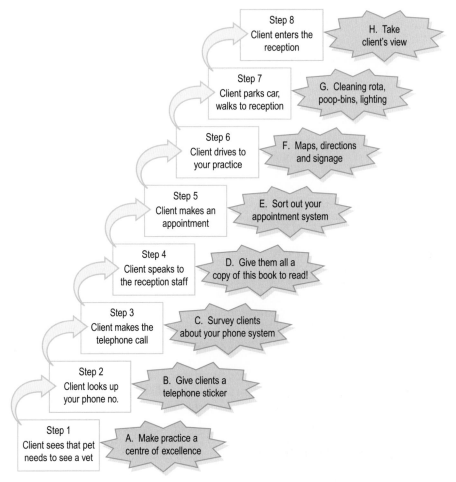

Figure 1.7   The various ways that a practice might improve the process of making an appointment and getting the client to the practice – to help the client on to the next step!

3. Ever phoned your practice – just like a client does? Are there particularly busy times of the day? Why not let your regular clients know the worst time to call when the lines are too busy? For every one that does phone outside these times, there'll be one less call to add to the chaos at peak times. Also, agreeing a practice protocol on what to do when the receptionist is unable to take the next incoming call will improve client relations tremendously.

4. All practice staff should have client care training (and support from the managers) so that they can do their best for the client.

5. As clients become more demanding, the practice needs to look at ways to adapt their working practices to become better at getting and keeping clients – with flexible working today, it is possible to improve services without adding to the costs.

6. Could you direct clients from far afield, whatever direction they are coming from? Even if you can't, I suspect someone in the practice can. So why not get it all written down, printed up and sealed to reception behind some clear plastic. Then, whoever answers the phone, even the new 'temp' at the weekend, will not have any problem giving directions using recognized landmarks, road names, numbers and so forth. Maps on-line and 'sat-nav' may be a help today, too. Also, look for improved signage to the practice; even local councils might consider a 'generic' sign 'Vet Clinic' if you suggest that drivers with sick animals in their cars need help in finding their way and councils want to keep roads safe, don't they!

7. There is no substitute, if you have a car park, for keeping it clean. Why not invest in 'poop-bins', sponsored and emptied by the practice, one each side of the practice along the road: it gives a strong message about responsible pet ownership, too.

8. The author did visit a practice in North Yorkshire where the front door jammed in the winter giving the impression that the place was shut! So, do you have good reception signage, a welcoming entrance that reflects the quality of the veterinary services?

HOW CONSUMERS ARE INFLUENCED BY SERVICE QUALITY

As consumers, when we purchase goods, there are three main deciding factors that we look at:

- Price – or the 'cost' to us of ownership
- Product quality – what we see as 'value' in the item
- Service quality – plus the 'convenience' or simplicity of getting the item.

Beyond this level of service quality, there is a further intangible differentiation, that of our overall 'experience' repeated over time bringing a longer-term relationship between us and the provider.

Where competing products appear the same then, for us, price is the deciding factor. If price is broadly similar then the next deciding level is product quality and, if price and product quality are pretty much the same (or we don't know enough about the technical aspects of the product to differentiate), then the quality of service that is associated with the product is used to select it. Repeat the purchase and our lifetime, user-friendly relationship has the *potential* to build our loyalty. Consider your local pub or restaurant where you have been visiting many times such that you get well-known by the bar staff or waiters. Your experience as a regular has the potential to be better than that of the casual visitor – it is human nature to build such relationships (Table 1.1 and Figure 1.8).

The *generic* product is what the client wants to buy – they want to buy milk, or pet food, or a flea treatment. Your local pub has *generic* walls and a ceiling – just like any other.

The *enhanced* product is the benefits the product will bring: skimmed milk may appeal as it is lower fat and seen to be better than whole milk; a pet food may be a slimming diet or low sodium; a systemic (injected) flea treatment may

Table 1.1   Deciding factors in product purchase

Product	Generic	Enhanced	Augmented	Potential
Pet food	Price per kg	Dog or cat? Flavour variety	Pet health management Vet endorsement Advertising	Weight monitoring Life stages advice Information on new diets
Flea treatment	Price	Topical Systemic Duration of cover	Professional advice Treating the home, too	New product innovations New indications Seasonal forecasts

be more effective than a topical (on the skin) treatment. Your local is open at *expected* times and serves usual beers and lagers.

The *augmented* product is everything related to what is being sold. It includes service, word of mouth references and convenience of locality for purchase, the market image of the product, and so on. Only about 20% of people make their buying decision based on price alone. The remaining 80% consider the value and benefits of the purchase as well as the price. Your local has a particularly good chef or bar staff, or your local independent brewery ales – the *augmented* offering.

The *potential* offering builds the relationship over time. Your milkman (or woman) may be able to respond to your varying demands as your social arrangements change (with family coming to stay, going on holiday, etc.) and build up a way to better serve your individual needs. Pet foods may similarly change over time. Or your local pub chef prepares gluten-free diets or special meals 'off-menu' for disabled clients who don't want to eat at usual opening times. (The author's local does – does yours?)

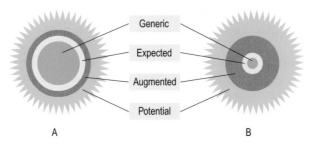

Generic
Expected
Augmented
Potential

A   B

Figure 1.8   Traditional strategic thinking Figure 8A provides a 'generic' offering, like every other practice focusing on the basic product or service where price comparisons are common. Compare this to the practice in Figure 8B; this practice offers an improved offering by focusing on the 'augmented' and 'potential' rings – those things that make a real difference to clients, keeping them loyal to the practice, and which they'll probably *pay more for!*

So, what about your practice? Does it focus on the generic product, like Figure 1.8a? Here, the focus is on the generic offering – products at the right price. The effective practice of tomorrow will pay attention to the service added offering by the 'augmented' and 'potential' rings (Figure 1.8b).

If one were to ask clients to veterinary practice what they consider to be the most important factors they think about when choosing veterinary services (or ranking), price or value for money tend to be the first thing mentioned. They will then probably go on to mention the veterinary surgeon, the welcome given by the practice staff, the accessibility of the practice (location) and of veterinary staff (availability of appointments with their chosen vet). When asked to *rate* their responses (score the relative importance of each issue from most to least important), while price is often first mentioned it often ends up around third on their list of importance behind the relationship with their vet, the welcome given by other staff, accessibility and availability, clarity of information, responsiveness and so forth. (Remember that list of determinants of general service quality described earlier where price did not feature. The next section deals with the determinants of service quality in veterinary practice specifically.)

If one were to look at a graph showing the relationship of increasing quality over time one would get something like Figure 1.9.

While in Figure 1.9a, the veterinary practice service delivery is continually increasing, it lags behind client expectation and they remain dissatisfied. In the second situation (Figure 1.9b), the practice has improved its service delivery now to exceed expectation and they have gained an advantage over other providers of animal health care. (Other providers include neighbouring practices as well as the pet superstore, animal health traders, the local pet shop, advice from breeders, or Joe down the pub!)

So, in today's competitive market, service quality is becoming more and more the deciding factor in purchasing goods. It is also becoming very significant in the purchase of services – and that includes veterinary services. There is no end-point with the search for quality service – it is a goal that can always be improved upon.

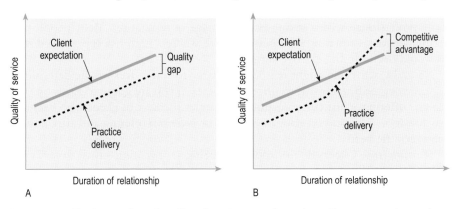

Figure 1.9 The interaction of quality of service over time when client expectation and practice delivery are compared showing how falling behind a client's expectation leads to a quality gap (a) while exceeding a client's expectations (b) can give a practice a competitive advantage over its rivals

HOW CLIENTS ASSESS VETERINARY SERVICE

Assessment of the level of veterinary services involves a number of factors of variable importance to the client:

People in the practice. Clients often buy 'people' rather than 'the service', because people are more *tangible*. In hiring the right people to work in reception in veterinary practice you, if you are a supervisor or head receptionist, or your partners, need to ensure recruits are people-orientated, friendly personalities and good communicators with experience in dealing with people and their problems. (For a modern guide on Recruitment, see Mackay (2007a).) They also need appropriate training for them to do their job well. You can see that whatever their technical expertise, the same criteria ought to be applied to clinical staff – nurses or assistant veterinary surgeons! (Unfortunately, veterinary surgeons are in ever-short supply!)

Level of quality. Quality measurement is important and necessary (see defining quality and service cycles, above).

Level of professional fees. Clients equate quality with a premium price, for example, Fortnum & Mason, Marks & Spencer, and designer labels, so fees are an important method for clients to judge quality of services that they hold in high regard (i.e. those which are difficult for them to evaluate directly). This assessment is based not so much on what they actually pay as what *value* they perceive from the payment.

In the author's experience, some clients do not understand why veterinary services cost as much as they do. One client was arguing with a recent graduate veterinary surgeon about the cost of a bitch spay. The vet explained that it took years of study to enable him to become qualified to do the surgery. The client replied that he had his City & Guilds as an electrician and he knew what professional services should cost! (A veterinary surgeon friend once observed that if you wanted an electric cooker fitted to your 30 amp ring main then get a vet to do it as they would charge less for a house call than an electrician!)

High fees often reflect a high self-image in the practice, and are often accepted from professionals with a strong positive image or reputation. Many people prefer higher fees – equating it to better service where a high risk is perceived such as would occur during elective surgery.

Naturally, what one might reasonably charge for one's fees will be determined to some degree by competitive prices. However, if you are going to focus on your *generic* offering – just cut your prices to attract the sort of client who wants to pay low fees or refocus on your *augmented* or *potential* offering and attract those who seek the best!

Waiting time. Clients do not appreciate being kept waiting – their time is valuable to them. Where a wait is necessary, for example if the veterinary surgeon is unavoidably held up with an emergency, informing the client what is happening and giving them the option of waiting or rebooking shows that the practice understands their time is valuable too.

Medical and surgical facilities. The medical and surgical facilities in the practice are part of the service to clients. Of course, if clients are not informed about them (see Chapter 3), they cannot appreciate them. A practice laboratory, for example, is often not cheaper to run than sending samples to a commercial laboratory, but has the major advantage of providing a rapid interpretation service to clients and is available for evening emergency work if the duty vet needs it.

Practice promotions. The way the practice markets itself and communicates its services to its clients is part of the differentiation process that helps clients choose between practices.

BUILDING THOSE INTANGIBLES

We saw that client service can be expressed in four levels, referred to as generic, enhanced, augmented and potential product. These are service circles (see Figure 1.8). The circle on the inside represents the generic or core expectations or needs of the client and will be pretty much the same as the next practice down the road. The next circle is the enhanced or perceptible level of service which, again, is something that your competitors are doing. The outer circle represents the augmented product and where client service begins to differentiate. However, it is the outer level or potential level that will differentiate the best practices of tomorrow. And remember, these perceptions are largely intangible. For most people, coming to the 'vet' is a necessity, not a pleasure. The purpose of striving for the outer augmented or potential level of service is to make the visit a highly satisfactory experience; the client's perceptions of the service received should be greater than their expectations (see Figure 1.8b).

Generic core level: fundamental client needs

In general terms, most clients come to a veterinary practice to, in no particular order:

■ speak with experts on the care of their animal.
■ get confirmation that they are doing the right thing for their pet.
■ off-load concerns about their animal's health and welfare.

Now, all practices provide this service to some degree and these factors provide the basis or generic core of veterinary service.

Expected level of service: the 'must-haves'

This is the standard of client service offered by the majority of practices. Appointment times, telephone response, message handling, sound records and accurate bills form the sort of thing that clients recognize as key service indicators. A practice must get these right – they are a 'given'.

Augmented service: 'raise your game'

An increasing number of veterinary practices compete at the higher or augmented service level. It is an opportunity for practice members really to use their imagination to create exceptional service for clients. Practices functioning at the augmented level are taking veterinary practice out of the basic commodity level and moving it towards a specialized or branded level. In product terms, it is like comparing generic-label products with brand-name products. Some people will seek the generic-label product, like own-label baked beans, others will seek the brand-name product, like Heinz beans, because of its association with quality and value. Many companies spend heavily on advertising to establish and maintain these brand values. The more the practice can differentiate itself through various initiatives to enhance its quality of service, the more control it has over its own development and progress (see Table 1.1).

And since a practice's staff become the brand – do you pay the minimum wage or attract the best staff that are properly trained and rewarded for the best service?

How to build a potential service: six ideas

How can you make a client's visit to your practice especially memorable and pleasant?

Even if you feel your service is better or more sophisticated than your rival, if clients don't see the difference, they will go back to their basic practices' criteria of evaluation and compare you on a fee basis – and the cheapest fees usually win.

You may already be doing these, but here are some ideas we've seen on our visits to practices across the country. Can you add to this list:

1. Fresh flowers in the waiting room.
2. Client loo checked and cleaned hourly.
3. Something for client's children to do quietly while they wait.
4. A free call to a local taxi firm that takes pets.
5. Thank-you notes, get well cards, a phone call a month after stitches out: 'how's she doing?'
6. Photos of clients and their pets to celebrate a successful case history.

BARRIERS TO EXCELLENCE

It is a sad fact of business life that there are many people who will find a reason to say what can't be done rather than ask 'why not?'. There are six major difficulties many practices face when trying to provide the best service to their clients:

1. Disagreement among the practice principals about the importance and value of quality client service.
2. General undervaluing of the client or, worse still, undervaluing the pet.
3. Failure to listen to clients. Too many veterinary surgeons believe they know what service their clients want when only the client knows what they really want.
4. Indifferent, unmotivated employees. Where there is little training, empowerment or motivation for delivering service quality excellence, staff do not see the value of the extra effort involved. If staff feel they are not valued they see little reason to value the client.

5. Frontline contact staff are powerless to solve most client's problems. Most clients will stay with the practice if their problem can be resolved immediately. By training and empowering front-line staff to deal with problems – and potential problems – client satisfaction will be much greater.
6. Practice dishonesty. There are many practices that claim to give good client service but really don't. Quality client service requires vigorous attention to detail. If the practice sets itself up to be the best practice in town, it has to be the best practice in town – at everything. It has to be the cleanest, smartest and most efficient practice, have the best staff, the best facilities, and so on. Clients soon notice if the fees charged are not, in their view, compatible with the service they receive – and they will go elsewhere.

PLANNING FOR EXCELLENCE IN CLIENT SERVICE

The aims when planning for excellence in client service are:

- To position yourself in a high-quality market niche.
- To develop a high-quality reputation within that niche.
- Constantly to manage your image.
- To concentrate your resources across a narrow front – that is, stick with the business you know best and don't try to diversify too much.
- To commit the practice to achieving better outcomes – make your clients so pleased with the caring service they receive that they want to come back *and* tell others about you. It is free marketing!

The first three points all deal with the practice image: how clients perceive the practice. Remember that their perception is their reality and that is what one needs to focus on. It is not enough simply to state that you have a high-quality practice – clients have to see *and* experience that too. Managing the practice image means constant attention to detail and constant sensitivity to client needs, and that requires the management of the practice to give the commitment to those ends. It does not happen just because someone says it should. Lack of commitment to constancy makes today's top practices tomorrow's mediocre ones. By concentrating on the business you know best and not trying to diversify too much, you have more control over what the practice achieves. Clients who are highly satisfied with the outcome of their visit will be very willing to come back again and again.

VALUING THE CLIENT

Clients don't care how much you know until they know how much you care.

Client service can only begin when the practice accepts that it is a client-driven business; that clients, and their animals, are essential to its survival. Veterinary surgeons, however, can sometimes be more interested in developing the intellectual and technical aspects of their craft than in being responsive to clients. All too often clients are regarded as rather annoying – and ignorant – interruptions to the day!

Earlier we gave a 10-point code of attitude to clients. So how do we achieve this?

THE PLAN OF ACTION

The aims cannot be achieved without a detailed plan of action. This plan can be broken down into 10 steps:

1. Commitment by head receptionists supported by practice leaders, principals or managers.
2. Identifying client needs.
3. Internal evaluation of the practice strengths and weaknesses in association with client service.
4. Setting goals and performance measures.
5. Putting the client's needs first.
6. Staff motivation.
7. Empowerment and training.
8. Assessing feedback.
9. Recognition and rewards.
10. Constant monitoring.

It is said that plans are nothing but that planning is all. In other words, the written plan means very little unless it is based upon a thorough understanding of what the practice stands for and can deliver, and its clients' needs. The thought processes involved in thinking through each step and involving all practice staff to put forward ideas to improve the service is, by itself, one of the most fruitful activities that the practice can consider from time to time.

So, let us take each in turn and look at key issues that need to be addressed to make the plan work. Naturally, there are some things that the management of the practice must do and these are recognized as possibly being outside the immediate control of the practice receptionist. However, the information is given, nonetheless, to provide a fuller picture of how to drive the customer service initiatives forward. Let us take each in turn.

COMMITMENT BY HEAD RECEPTIONISTS

Focusing on clients is not simply a case of coming up with a new wish-list of intent about client care. It involves change and commitment in the practice's whole attitude starting with that of the senior partners. They are responsible for setting standards, modelling behaviour, committing resources, and communicating their full support and commitment to everyone. And they always have to stay involved. As head receptionist, it is essential to 'walk what you talk'; to lead by example. Telling your junior staff that you are committed to your clients, whereas in reality you ignore them and are rude about them behind their backs gives a dishonest message and will encourage your staff to behave in the same way. On the other hand, answering the phone appropriately yourself, helping an older client to the car, or wiping down a dirty wall when your staff are busy, and praising your staff when you see them doing a good job, encourages your staff to follow your example of commitment to service.

IDENTIFYING CLIENT NEEDS

Reality to your clients is the way they see things. Their perception equates to their reality. To get a clear picture of their perception, ask them:

- Why they come to you for their animal care needs?
- What do they value about the services and products in your practice?
- What do they like about the practice?
- What would they change if they were running the practice?
- How do you compare to your competitors?
- What would they want you to stop doing?
- What would they want you to do more of to please them?

(See Research techniques for client feedback, in Chapter 4.)

Experience has shown that today's veterinary clients of pet animals want some fundamental services:

- Full animal health care for their pets – a one-stop-shop.
- Quality service that they define.
- Easy access to the veterinary surgeon (which may mean offering more flexible hours in the clinic).
- Behaviour services (behaviour problems are the primary cause of euthanasia in young animals).
- Diagnostic services.
- Dental services (including preventive care advice).

How many of these are you providing in your practice? How do your clients' needs differ?

Having got the fundamentals right every time – what can you do to *augment* your service and raise your game to *potential* services?

INTERNAL EVALUATION OF PRACTICE STRENGTHS AND WEAKNESSES

By identifying what you are (or are not) doing currently for your clients, you know where you are starting from before improving your service to clients.

To do things right means:

- Finding out what your clients' require (see section on assessing client feedback in Chapter 4).
- Specifying what those requirements mean practically.
- Identifying key indicators or measures that you can track to learn which requirements are met and which are not. So, a key requirement for clients might be a maximum 15 minutes waiting time for a 10-minute consult frequency. Does your current system achieve this? If not, how can you modify it to reduce waiting time to an acceptable level?

SETTING GOALS AND PERFORMANCE MEASURES

Having done an internal assessment of what is going on in the practice, and an external assessment of your clients' needs, the results must be integrated to develop the goals and performance measures for client service in the practice.

Goals should be clear, simple and easy to measure; they should also be prominently placed in the practice for all to see including, where appropriate, your clients. For example, if you are working to improve your telephone services (see Chapter 5), tell your clients. If you introduce a new service such as better laboratory facilities, tell your clients. Help them see and understand you are constantly striving to improve your overall service to them; show them that they matter to you. This may encourage them to be more forthcoming on how well you are achieving the goals you set.

Do not try to do too much at once, as it can be confusing and overwhelming. Bigger goals, for example, can be broken into smaller, simpler stages. However, do not strive for less than 100% quality service; 90% quality is not acceptable. Consider a midwife who works at 90% quality performance ('she only drops one in ten babies!'), or a chauffeur driving at 80% quality performance ('He only hit one in five cars today!') – no more acceptable than your practice striving for less than 100% quality.

PUTTING THE CLIENTS' NEEDS FIRST

The change from a work-driven culture to a client-driven culture is very big. It means putting the needs of the client (and their pet) first. Identify client needs by asking them what they'd like – then act on it. For example, if you only have a modest car park, then why do you let staff park their cars there? OK, so you may have concerns about leaving your practice late in the evening – but do you all do that? Veterinary surgeons going in and out throughout the day have a clear need to park close to the practice. But remember the number of clients who visit each day with an animal that they cannot carry yet who has a problem walking.

The author visited a practice in SE London to run a receptionist's training course the next day. He witnessed an elderly German shepherd dog, too big to carry yet obviously lame, have to walk from the car parked round the corner as the car park was full. The next day, one junior receptionist said that she chose to work there so she could park her car right outside where she worked (so she could keep an eye on it) and couldn't see the need to move it. Perhaps she was in the wrong job!

STAFF MOTIVATION

Client relations mirror employee relations. It is important that all staff consistently give the caring image you would like if you were a client of the practice. The way staff are treated is the way they will treat clients. When a client meets a staff member, they are the practice for the client. Making sure you get practice information to your colleagues in reception, such as monthly income, food sales targets, and progress towards goals, helps keep everyone involved and interested.

By letting them feel an important part of the practice, they will be more motivated to help clients. See Mackay (2007b) for some useful and practical advice on staff motivation.

EMPOWERMENT AND TRAINING

You and your colleagues need training and empowering to do the best for clients. This means you should have the right to make your own decisions to help clients. (See Chapter 8 for ideas about finding client solutions. For example, although it may be a practice policy to have a strict policy on refunds, do you have the power to flex the rules on refunds against clear guidelines for certain situations?)

ASSESSING CLIENT FEEDBACK

Face-to-face interviews, random phone calls and short questionnaires handed out in the waiting room are three easy methods to ascertain your current level of client service right from the horse's mouth – the clients themselves.

Negative comments and criticisms are nothing to fear. They provide specific opportunities for you to improve your service. Negative comments may include client complaints like the pet being returned smelly after a day in hospital, being kept waiting a long time for an appointment, difficulty contacting the practice by phone, not getting a space in your car park because of staff cars, or difficult access for disabled people. Often clients are too polite to say them directly to you. Many of these problems can be resolved quickly. But what about complaints about 'staff attitude', 'tone of voice on the telephone', being 'unhelpful', and so on? These grey areas can be more difficult to measure and correct, but it is possible and it is very important.

The process of assessing client satisfaction should be repeated regularly. By keeping constantly in touch with the clients' level of satisfaction you can nip problems in the bud and give prompt feedback to your staff. This is a key area and one worth contracting specialist help – go to www.daw.co.uk for some professional advice with experience of the veterinary sector.

RECOGNITION AND REWARDS

Part of effective motivation is rewarding and recognizing when people have done a good job or come up with an innovative and exciting idea. Reward can be anything from a simple 'Thank you' to a cash bonus, but it should be open to everyone. One of the better rewards that people often appreciate is time off – say leaving half an hour early one evening or having a longer lunch-break (or one at all!) carries a good feeling and does not actually upset the practice finance too much. Encouraging staff members to congratulate each other also helps a team to work together.

CONSTANT MONITORING

It is not enough to set up a service improvement system and then leave it. It needs constant reassessment and monitoring to remain truly effective and ahead of the competition. Go back to the key stages discussed in Figures 1.5–1.7 – you are aiming to keep the client on track and not fall through the rungs!

WHAT ABOUT THE QUALITY OF HEALTH CARE?

> Health care is not a Product or a simple service that can be standardized, packaged, marketed, or adequately judged by consumers according to quality and price.
> A. Relman, Professor of Medicine and of Social Medicine, Harvard Medical School

Although quality and quality service have been dealt with fairly extensively in this first chapter, it is important not to lose sight of the fact that a veterinary surgeon's prime role is, and always will be, treating and caring for animals. Veterinary medical care is a highly personal and individualized service, the true value and success of which can be fully appreciated only by individuals in their individual circumstances.

> Business managers don't understand why they shouldn't be able to get reliable information about quality of care, which they can weigh against the prices charged. The fact is that the measurement of quality is in a primitive state and is likely to remain so for the foreseeable future. Here is the best definition of high quality medical care that I can come up with: it is the care given to a particular patient under particular circumstances by a compassionate and competent physician who has access to consultants and the best current information, who is not influenced by economic incentives to do more or less than is medically appropriate, and who is committed to serve the patient's best interests guided by the latter's wishes and medical needs. This definition emphasizes the physician's key role in allocating medical resources and presenting standards of quality.
>
> A. Relman, Professor of Medicine and of Social Medicine, Harvard Medical School

The quote from Mr Relman is equally applicable to the practice of veterinary medicine. It is difficult to quantify, but it should never be devalued by greed or selling unnecessary services.

CONCLUSION

Achieving excellence in client service is like people's desire to stop smoking or to lose weight. They know and want the goal, they know how to do it, and they know it's worth doing, but they don't like putting up with the temporary discomfort to achieve a long-term goal. Client service is not 'frill', nor is it merely problem solving, so education and training of staff alone is not adequate. Helping people achieve the aim of excellence in client service means helping them find the self-discipline they need. This means that a well thought-out programme or system is necessary. Developing a monitoring system in your practice may create short-term discomfort, and will certainly require disciplined changes in daily lifestyle, but it will encourage practice members to live up to the goals to which they have agreed, and give excellent client service.

> ### SUMMARY
> 1. Veterinary practice is a professional service business.
> 2. Client service is satisfying client needs.
> 3. Client service is the major distinguishing factor between practices for clients.
> 4. Client satisfaction = perception – expectation.
> 5. Quality is an integral part of excellent client service but is not always easy to measure.
> 6. Excellence in client service can be planned for.
>
> Having read this chapter, add some ideas for a Plan of Action in the Appendix. (Did you know, if you write it down, it is more likely to get done?!)

References

Mackay, A.R. (2007a) *Recruiting, Retaining, & Releasing People.* Butterworth Heinemann.

Mackay, A.R. (2007b) *Motivation, Ability & Confidence Building in People.* Butterworth Heinemann.

Chapter 2
Make your first impressions count

THOSE FIRST FEW SECONDS

As humans, we are extremely good at making judgements of situations or places in a matter of seconds. This probably goes back to the time when we wore animal skins and had to make quick decisions or run the risk of being eaten!

Your client may have had only a short conversation with you on the phone or their first visit to the practice, possibly about nothing in particular, but they will go away with a quite detailed impression of you and the practice. These first impressions will stay with them and colour their judgement, so we have to strive to get it right every time. In making this evaluation, they will be using many of their senses, sound, sight, smell and touch.

As the client's first point of contact with the practice, you will convey to them the practice's image, by your attitude, appearance and manner towards them. How many times have you been into a shop, looked around at the interior and the staff, then turned on your heel and walked out. Why? Because the shop looked tatty and the staff showed no interest in you. The same goes for the practice if a new client walks in, sees an untidy waiting room and someone behind the reception desk who is probably closely related to Attila the Hun. So what do they do – turn and walk out. They certainly are not going to trust a valued member of their family to such a place.

Why your job is so important is that, as the practice's representative, you never get a second chance to make a first impression. Remember that each client is different. *First impressions are the ones that last.* Here are some basic rules that will help to build those first impressions.

1. Look at your client as soon as they walk in. Make eye contact, acknowledge their arrival, even if you are on the phone, or dealing with another client or colleague.
2. Focus on them, almost to the extent of ignoring what else is going on around you, very hard to do in a busy reception. Pay attention to what they are doing and saying. Make a fuss of their pet, and use the animal's name.
3. Smile. A smile costs you nothing, yet it can generate a large amount of warmth and well being towards the client, and you will feel better in yourself. A word of warning – don't overdo the smile, as this will appear false, insincere and very patronizing. It will also put the client on their guard and make them

think, 'why are they smiling at me like that, are they trying to cover up something, am I dealing with an idiot?' Also, be conscious of your body language (see non-verbal communication, p. 38).

THOSE 'MOMENTS OF TRUTH'

Tom Peters, a renowned management guru from America, suggested the idea of 'Moments of Truth'. This means no matter what your Yellow Pages advertisement says about you, or what your boss may say about looking after clients, it comes down to those individual moments of contact that a client has with your practice that become a 'moment of truth' about the practice and its service. And those moments of truth are never more important than in those first moments of contact.

Put yourself on the other side of the reception desk. If you were a client visiting or telephoning your practice for the first time, what might *your* expectations be in the following circumstances:

- During a first phone call?
- On a first visit?

During a first phone call, you would probably expect the greeting from the receptionist to be polite and not to keep you waiting. And apologize if you were kept waiting. You would hope that they had all the right information to hand, took a message clearly, or put you through swiftly to the right person. You would expect to be politely questioned so that the practice got the right details of what you wanted, were not treated in an off-hand manner, and were listened to. Conversations should be pleasant and impart accurate information. It may be necessary for the practice veterinary surgeon to call you back, or take details so that they can send information to you. They should end the phone call politely and offer you further help or advice if you contact them. Following the phone call, you might expect the practice to make the necessary arrangements so that, when you did visit, they were expecting you and had your pet booked in.

When you visited the practice for the first time you would expect the reception area to be clean and bright, tidy and not 'smell'. You would expect the products to be displayed attractively and information easy to read. As far as the staff are concerned, you would expect them all to be professional, appropriately dressed, helpful, readily available, quick to serve and prompt to communicate. You would expect them to know what they are doing and to be able to solve problems in a reasonable time – or find someone who can. You would expect to be kept informed about what is going on and treated as an individual. You would hope that they would see any problems you or your pet had as an opportunity to demonstrate what the practice could do to put it right.

Then you would hope that your experiences of their service – or the products you bought from them – would reinforce those first impressions. It is all these tiny events and experiences that go together to make up those crucial 'moments of truth' for you. One thing going wrong can spoil the whole experience for you and put you off going back – unless the practice can recover brilliantly!

Chapter 5 will look at telephone skills in more depth and it is a very important chapter. Get the telephone communication wrong and you may never have the opportunity to do anything for that owner's pet, as they will not bring it in to see you. However, assuming that you get that right and the owner does come in, then when they arrive and park their car – as most owners will arrive by car, so few actually live within walking distance – the ease of parking will be their next moment of truth. You may not be able to do much about the car park – except make sure it is kept clean (and free of staff cars! See page 22) – but you do have an opportunity to make a real impact at the next moment of truth: when the client opens the door and steps into the waiting room.

THE WAITING ROOM

Consider the waiting room to be the shop window of the practice. What it looks like will greatly affect whether the client actually comes over the threshold and speaks to you. Coming through the waiting room area will be a journey of the senses: sight, smell, taste, touch and hearing. This journey will tell the client a tremendous amount about the practice. It will give them a good idea about the practice's attitude and professionalism.

Are the posters on the walls old and tattered or up to date? Do they flutter in the breeze when the door is opened? Do they convey some of the practice's values, such as the importance of preventive healthcare programmes and first class veterinary care, or are they just there to cover up the cracks and the faded paint-work? With the new Medicine Regulations 2006, please remember that these posters must not promote a Prescription Only Medicine – Veterinarian (POM-V) or Prescription Only Medicine – Veterinarian, Pharmacist, Suitably Qualified Person (POM-VPS) product, though if you have a separate reception area for Farmers then posters for this category of products may be displayed.

Do the notices on the notice board go back to when the practice was started? Lost a black cat, May 1965. Are the notices written or neatly typed? Are they set out in a logical fashion or just jumbled up? Do you regularly check the cards?

Is the seating clean and smart, or does it look as if it's just been taken out of a skip; are the covers patched up with sticky plaster? Is the floor clean, or is it covered with animal hair and looking more like a back street barber's shop. Worst of all, does the place smell of urine or faeces, or does it have a clean hospital environment smell.

Are the shelves of the display cabinet stacked neat and tidy, with dog and cat food or are the bags split and dirty, and are the shelves about to break under the strain?

How often do you walk through the waiting room when you arrive for work, look at it through the client's eyes? Do you like what you see? Do you feel welcome? Does what you see convey a sense of professionalism? Ask yourself, would you be happy bringing a member of your family into such an environment? If your answer is 'no' to any of these questions, then do something about it and quick. If you don't have to go through the waiting reception area, make sure you periodically check the 'front of house' appearance. Be objective in your appraisal, because if you are not, that new or prospective client may not even make it to the desk!

Felt boards for notices, divide into subjects:

Lost & Found, Important Health Information, Wanted, Forthcoming Events, i.e. Puppy parties.

Checklist:

- Front door opens easily
- Smell
- Posters
- Floor clean
- Chairs tidy and clean
- Notices up to date
- Reception desk tidy and accessible.

ATTITUDE

If you can remain friendly, *all* the time, you're most of the way there. It may mean doing some shouting and screaming when you're out of sight and earshot. One practice keeps all its chipped coffee mugs for staff to throw at the large metal dustbins at the back of the surgery to work off steam. Well, it is certainly better than taking it out on the next client.

If you can add cheerfulness to friendliness, and maybe a bit of enthusiasm, when appropriate, it's going to be easier to cope with the pet-owning public. If you are actually helpful into the bargain, then there is not a lot anyone will be able to complain about. To do all this with calmness and efficiency will put you in the 'super' league.

Difficult? Every day, all the time, whatever the weather, and whatever the problems at home, or in the operating theatre? Of course it's difficult. However, put yourself in the client's shoes. What sort of person would you like to meet when you need help?

DRESS

Is what you are wearing appropriate? Above all, you need to be dressed appropriately for the job. This may mean wearing a uniform, or it may not but, to look professional, your clothes must fit the work you are doing.

Consider when making a choice:

The colour: colours that show every spot of blood, or worse, are very difficult to maintain all the work period.

Material: the material your clothes are made of also matters. If it is something that picks up every dog or cat hair, it's going to need a lot more time to keep it clean. However, if it's easily brushable, it will leave you more time for looking after your clients.

Footwear: shoes need to be comfortable, of course. They need to be smart. Trainers, though comfortable, do not look particularly professional. As your appearance is a vital part of your job, ask your practice if they are prepared to give you a clothes allowance, to help keep you looking smart.

Identification: it is important your clients know who you are and your role within the practice. It is very much easier for a client to communicate with you and easier for you to respond and it maintains a friendlier atmosphere. There is nothing more frustrating than to tell someone your problem in detail, only to find you've been talking to the wrong person. Most service organizations make sure their staff wear a name badge. What you put on the badge is also important; if you are security conscious and do not want everyone knowing your forename or surname, then a job title together with the name of the practice will be sufficient.

WHAT TO DO BEFORE YOU ANSWER THE PHONE

Before you can answer the phone, there are certain procedures that you need to go through in order to create the right impression (see Chapter 5, Telephone skills).

As with the first few seconds of visual impression when the client walks into the practice, the audio picture is also important. So, if you follow this basic checklist, you won't go far wrong.

- Phone in a convenient position. For right- and left-handed users.
- Pencil and pen by the phone. For some reason, pens have a habit of disappearing – try using pens with a chain attached! It is amazing how many pens some colleagues can collect.
- Do not rely on scraps of paper to record any messages or information. Use either a day book/diary or a dedicated messages book. There are books on the market that have carbonless paper, so you have a copy and the recipient has the top copy of any message. Useful for checking to see if the message has been actioned. Or get it on the computer immediately.

Do have a checklist of questions that you need to ask callers if they phone requesting an appointment or advice.

This is for two reasons:

1. If you get as much information down over the phone as you can, it will save time when the client arrives in the surgery.
2. If there were ever a dispute or complaint from a client, bearing in mind the litigious times we live in, about advice or information given on the phone, you can refer to your records.

Basic questions for that checklist: use this as a guide and devise your own:

- How long has the animal been ill?
- Has it been sick?
- Is it bleeding, and from where?

- Is it on any medication?
- When did it last eat?
- Can you bring it in immediately?
- Where is it located, in the case of equine clients.

A LASTING IMPRESSION

- How will the client remember their visit?
- Will they remember the bill, or the way you helped them with their visit?
- Was your attitude towards them positive?
- What will they remember?
- The last impression or exit is just as important as that first impression, get the exit wrong and you may never see that client again.

Here are some ideas:

- Commenting on the product they have chosen, and personally recommending it if you have used it.
- Commenting on their good choice (not too obviously).
- Offering to hold their pet while they write out the cheque or credit card slip.
- Using the client's name.
- Talking to the client's children.
- Holding the door open as they leave the waiting room.

And finally:

Those crucial 'moments of truth' can occur at that first telephone contact right through to the client departing the practice – and anywhere in between! Make sure that all those contacts lead along a strong chain of excellent client service. And remember, a chain is only as strong as its weakest link. This book aims to ensure that you find ways to strengthen all those links wherever you have an influence.

Chapter 3
Focus on your client

The client is the most important person to your practice, they pay your salary and without them you have no job, so it is very important how you treat them. This chapter deals with how to focus on them so they feel that they are the only client – the *numero uno*.

FOCUS ON THE FACE-TO-FACE

Communication between two human beings, whatever their relationship to each other, is a complex process. Face-to-face communication is potentially the best and clearest method of sending and receiving messages and information. However, as it is so complex, it is often fraught with problems – there are more ways for things to go wrong.

COMMUNICATION AT WORK

Good communication skills are essential in a work environment where efficiency is dependent on the speed and effectiveness of the exchange of information of all kinds. Keeping the lines of communication clear of misunderstandings, as far as possible, is one way of ensuring high productivity and encouraging teamwork.

Communication objectives

There are four main objectives behind every communication task. The *sender* of the message or signal wants to be:

- heard
- understood
- accepted and
- initiate action, or a change of thinking, behaviour or attitude in the receiver.

This is regardless of any other objectives there may be, such as to inform, entertain, explain, convince, persuade or sympathize.

If any of the four major objectives are not achieved, then it leads to frustration. To avoid this eventuality, it is essential, as sender, first, to know exactly what you want to say and, second, to say it as clearly as possible. As the receiver, it is important to listen as actively as possible.

Communication is both sending and receiving messages

Communication goes on continually whenever two people are together. All of it is important and whether you are conscious of it or not, you react and respond to it. It pays to be aware of yourself and of other people's methods of communicating.

LISTENING

Even though listening is a key communication skill, we often find listening with our full attention is something that is quite difficult to do.

This is because, every day, the average person is bombarded with thousands of messages in the form of both spoken and written words. We receive messages as:

- face-to-face conversations
- telephone conversations
- overheard conversations
- newspapers and magazines
- letters
- bills, reminders, parking tickets, junk mail
- radio
- television
- billboards and other large advertising displays.

If we were to pay full attention to every message that is directed towards us we would have brain overload. So, instead of paying full attention, we tend to filter out most of the incoming messages and only really listen to those that we perceive as important for us. For example, if you have the TV on at home while you are reading or writing a letter, providing you are absorbed in your task, you will filter out the sound. But if a favourite programme comes on you will tune in to that and suddenly become aware of what you are missing, even though the volume on the TV set has not been turned up.

As a result, all of us are very good at *not listening*, and usually not so good at *listening*. We can easily fall into the habit of thinking:

'Oh no, I've heard this before!' or,

'I'm not interested in this' or,

'Here we go again!' or,

'I know about this, so I don't need to listen.'

We become passive rather than active listeners, which means that, when someone talks to us, we can easily switch off to concentrate on our own thoughts. Even though we may *give the appearance of listening*, we are actually paying very little attention either to the speaker, or what is being said.

Clearly, if someone is looking at the ceiling, yawning, continually checking their watch or looking away from you, then they are not listening and not paying attention.

When you are not being listened to you feel:

- angry
- irritated
- disappointed
- as though carrying on with the conversation would be a waste of time
- that you do not feel as though you want to listen to anything the other person has to say to you.

Obviously, if there is someone, either at work or at home, who consistently does not listen to you, then this is bound to have a bad effect on your relationship with them.

SWITCHING OFF

Even though the person speaking may be telling you something you do not want to hear, or something you disagree with, switching off or tuning them out will not help the situation. In fact, it will probably make matters worse because once they realize you are not listening they will become irritated and annoyed.

CONCENTRATING

Effective listeners concentrate on the message and really try to understand what is being said.

ASSUMING

Although it is often easy to assume we know what is coming next or that we have *heard it all before*, we can never be really sure. Making assumptions about what the speaker is going to say can be very dangerous, particularly when dealing with client complaints.

THINKING AHEAD

It is impossible simultaneously to concentrate on what is being said and think about what your reply will be. Effective listeners consider what they want to say only after the speaker has finished speaking.

DAYDREAMING

Daydreaming or just *giving the appearance* of listening is a waste of time and extremely unprofessional.

MENTALLY JUDGING AND/OR CRITICIZING

It is impossible to give the speaker your full attention if you are mentally judging or criticizing some aspect of what they are saying, or their appearance, personality or mannerisms.

FINISHING SENTENCES

Even when the speaker is long-winded, confusing or confused, effective listeners never interrupt, *talk over* or finish other people's sentences for them. It is tempting to finish people's sentences just to speed the conversation up. Yes, it can be difficult, but elective listening *is* hard work sometimes!

STATUS

Effective listeners pay equal attention to everyone and do not allow a person's status (regardless of whether the speaker is the senior partner of the practice or the most junior member of the team) to affect how well they listen.

The most important part of listening is concentrating. Here are some ideas to help you do this:

- *Be prepared to listen.* Start off on the right foot by giving the speaker the chance to put a point of view and be genuinely interested to hear it.
- *Be interested.* Look for ways that the message or point of view is relevant to you or your job.
- *Keep an open mind.* Be aware of your own prejudices and feelings, not only about the subject but also the speaker. You may hold strong views on, say, euthanasia, keep them to yourself. Don't jump to conclusions or you may miss an important point or message. Delay your judgement.
- *Listen for the main ideas.* Don't just hear the facts; sort out the principles and the drift of the argument from the detail. Try to prioritize what the client is saying to you, so when you summarize what they have told you and the action you are going to take it will come out in a logical order.
- *Listen critically.* Weigh up the value of the evidence and logic behind the main message.

TO SUMMARIZE EFFECTIVE LISTENING

Effective listening involves:

- Never making assumptions about what the speaker plans to say next.
- Never thinking ahead and framing your answer while someone is still speaking because, at that point, you have not heard the whole story.

- Never daydreaming or giving the appearance of listening.
- Never mentally judging or criticizing either the speaker themselves, or what they have to say. Never interrupting, jumping in or taking over.

LISTENING SKILLS

Do:

- Look at the speaker.
- Recognize the speaker's feelings and viewpoint.
- Look for points to agree with.
- Give brief summaries of what you have heard.
- Nod your head, make encouraging comments.
- Reserve judgement until you have all the information.

Don't:

- Interrupt the speaker.
- Start thinking about something else.
- Let your previous experience of the person put you off.
- Let your prejudices get in the way.
- Put down or ridicule the speaker or the subject.
- Change the subject.
- Fidget or distract the speaker.

QUESTIONING

Asking the right kinds of questions will often be the only way to find out:

- What the problem *really is*.
- What the client really wants you to do about it.

There are three types of questions – closed, leading and open – which can be asked. It is important that you understand the difference between them and know which kinds of questions should be used to gain the maximum amount of information.

CLOSED QUESTIONS

Closed questions generally invite a one-word, factual answer, most usually 'Yes' or 'No'. Some examples of closed questions are:

- Did you pay cash for this?

Answer 1: Yes

Answer 2: No

- Did you give it twice a day?

Answer 1: Yes

Answer 2: No

- Have you explained all this to the practice manager?
Answer 1: Yes
Answer 2: No.

Closed questions will not encourage the client to give you a great deal of information, and will generally not help very much trying to identify and solve a problem.

LEADING QUESTIONS

Leading questions should also be avoided because they suggest to the client that you expect a certain kind of answer. Leading questions will not help you to get to the root of the problem and may annoy clients. Some examples of leading questions are:

- I suppose you read the instructions, didn't you?
- Do you realize that it is to be given between meals?
- I don't suppose you washed your hands afterwards?
- You've had it a long time, haven't you?

OPEN QUESTIONS

Open questions generally begin with:

- How?
- Why?
- What?
- Who?
- When?
- Where?

They will provide you with the maximum amount of information. This is because they require the person being asked the question really to give the matter some thought. Some examples of open questions are:

- Whom did you speak to at the practice?
- When did you first notice the problem?
- How have you tried to use it?
- Why do you think that happens?
- Where does the fault seem to be?
- What exactly seems to be wrong with it?
- Whom have you spoken to about this so far?

By using good listening skills, open and friendly body language and by asking a range of open questions you should be able to find out:

- What the client thinks the problem is.
- The history of the problem.
- The current situation.
- What the client wants.

CHECKLIST

Effective questioning involves:

- Avoiding closed and leading questions.
- Using open questions which start with:
    How? Why? What? Who? When? Where?
    to gain as much information as possible.

NON-VERBAL COMMUNICATION

People cannot read your mind; they can only see your actions and hear your words.

The absence of words does not mean the absence of communication. Up to 90% of all communication is non-verbal; remember we talked with our bodies long before we had language.

Non-verbal communication is a wide-ranging and varied subject and, because it is not only multi-faceted but also subtle, it is not possible to draw up hard and fast rules. Gestures, expressions or tone of voice can be interpreted in many ways according to its juxtaposition with other kinds of communication signals, in another situation, in other cultures.

When you are dealing with a client face to face, how aware are you of the non-verbal signals you are sending? Do you respond to the signals sent to you? How can you utilize this information in your role as a communicator? Are there any non-verbal clues that you give out and which you would rather not do, for instance do you sound irritated and short-tempered when you are tired? Do you forget to smile or show appreciation of people at times?

Listed below are some examples of attitudes and how they are commonly expressed non-verbally in our culture. Try to make your own list using your own experience. The list is not definitive, but will give you a general idea.

Openness: A woman will have her hands down at her side. Men who are open and friendly will have their coats unbuttoned.

Defensiveness: The very young will cross or clasp their arms when defying their parents' instructions; the very old cross their arms when they want to be heard, and others cross their arms to isolate or protect themselves.

Evaluation: A person who strikes a pose with hand on cheek, stroking the chin, and cocking the head slightly to one side may be said to be evaluating a situation.

Rejection: The most obvious gestures of rejection are folding the arms, moving the body away, crossing the legs and tilting the head forward, the person either peering over his or her glasses or squinting as if trying to see what is said more clearly.

Doubt, suspicion, puzzlement: A person rubbing or touching his or her nose lightly with an index finger after being asked a question is expressing doubt or puzzlement. This gesture is usually accompanied by squirming in a chair, twisting the body into a silhouette position or physically withdrawing.

Reassurance: In adults, clenched hands with thumbs rubbing against each other is a common reassurance gesture.

Cooperation: A person sitting forward in his or her chair, feet on tiptoes, and tilting his or her head indicates that at least he or she is listening.

Confidence: Confident people have more frequent and longer lasting eye contact than those who are unsure. The confident person usually has a proud erect stance, makes a few hand-to-face gestures when speaking, and is inclined to make gestures with his or her hands.

Nervousness: This is expressed by gestures such as fidgeting in a chair, jingling money in pockets, tugging at trousers or dress while sitting, biting lip, and picking at fingernails.

Self-control: Holding an arm behind the back and clenching the hand tightly while the other hand grips the wrist or arm is a common gesture of self-control.

Acceptance: Moving closer to another person, thereby closing the gap between you, is an indicator of acceptance. Copying someone else's body position also demonstrates empathy and acceptance of the other person.

Honesty, credibility and sincerity: The palm is placed over the heart; a frown often means disapproval; a person who is lying often draws the index finger over the nostrils.

TIPS FOR NON-VERBAL COMMUNICATION

Messages and signals are communicated in many ways other than verbally.

Some of these are:

- Facial expression
- Eye contact
- Position of body
- Gestures
- Position in room in relation to other people
- Tone of voice
- Emphasis/speed/inflexions in voice
- Deliberate silence
- Timing
- Clothes/appearance
- Touch.

GETTING THE MESSAGE ACROSS

Do:

- Be clear about what you are saying – look at your listener(s).
- Speak clearly.
- Consider the listener's feelings.
- Choose the right time and place.
- Match your words with the way you say them.
- Check that the listener has understood.
- Vary the tone and pace of your voice.

Don't:

- Complicate the message with detail or jargon; talk so much that the listener cannot comment or ask questions.
- Be vague.
- Attack or ridicule your listener(s).
- State views on subjects you know will irritate.
- Ignore signs of confusion, resentment or lack of interest in your listeners(s).
- Put on an act, or exaggerate.
- Speak in a remote, detached way.

Look at your own body language, when you are talking to clients and colleagues and remember:

Positive body language, which shows that you are listening includes:

- Facing the other person.
- Leaning forwards towards the speaker, rather than away from them, and maintaining steady eye contact, but without staring.
- Nodding agreement.
- Smiling rather than scowling or frowning.
- Keeping a relaxed open posture and not fussing with pieces of paper or checking your watch.

Negative body language, which shows you are *not* listening includes:

- Turning away.
- Frowning, glaring or remaining impassive and 'stony-faced'.
- Leaning back, arms folded.
- Refusing to maintain eye contact, looking away or gazing over the speaker's head.
- Foot or pen tapping.
- Paper shuffling.

NON-VERBAL CHECKLIST

Try to match the non-verbal signals to the meanings in the list:

- a person turning their face away
- a person slumping in a chair
- a person shaking her head slowly
- a person facing you but with eyes down or looking away
- hands clenched tight
- a person sitting upright on the edge of a chair
- a deep breath
- pacing up and down
- a broad smile
- a loud voice
- shrugging shoulders
- a shaky hesitant voice

- fiddling with keys, change, bag
- a person sitting with arms folded legs crossed
- leaning back on chair, hands behind head.

Here is a list of suggested meanings:

1. Boredom, lack of interest, sulking
2. 'No, I don't think so' or 'Oh, no you don't'
3. Refusing to listen, upset
4. Lack of interest, guilt
5. Attentiveness or nervousness
6. Hostility, defensiveness
7. Tension, anxiety, nervousness
8. Shock, or the start of saying something difficult
9. Irritation, anxiety
10. Pleasure
11. Anger, dominance
12. Uncertainty, nervousness, fear
13. 'Don't know, don't care'
14. Tension, anxiety, irritation
15. Assurance, relaxation, superiority.

GIVING 110%

So what is this mythical 110% you are supposed to give clients?
   Excellent service is, in fact, giving the client a little more than they expect.
   It is:

- Looking interested and ready to help.
- Being flexible enough to drop what you are doing and help.
- Allowing clients to be right (even when they may not be).

If you can deliver what the client needs, then you will have a great deal of job satisfaction and clients will really enjoy coming to the practice.
   Add some ideas for action to your list in the Appendix.

Chapter 4
Making the client feel 'special'

Good service relies on the ability to make the client feel special. No one wants to feel that they are 'just another client'. Instead, everyone wants to feel that they are being treated as an individual.

The example (Box 4.1) was taken from a veterinary surgeon's own experience attending a doctor's clinic recently.

EVERY CLIENT IS UNIQUE

The term 'client' covers wide ranges of people. All of them are different and all of them want different kinds of service from you and the practice. Just because what you did for your last client was acceptable to them, do not assume that your next client will want the same. That said, there are some pretty fundamental things that all client's need, but not adapting the way we treat people to suit the particular circumstances means we run the risk of people feeling they are just a number.

Your skill lies in being able to get to the heart of the individual client quickly and understand what makes them tick. You can then satisfy – and exceed – their expectations of client service.

THE GOLDEN RULES FOR MAKING PEOPLE FEEL SPECIAL

Service Plus: this is an acronym for the following:

- *Positive* – clients expect you to take a positive view of them and addressing their needs.
- *Listening* – no matter how often you have 'seen it all before', each client views their situation and needs as unique.
- *Understanding* – this comes with experience and will be explored later. Suffice to say that there are both human and animal effects in any given situation that need be understood.
- *Showing it* – no matter what you may feel about a situation, none of your clients will be a good mind reader, so you will have to communicate your understanding and positive approach clearly to all types of client.

Box 4.1   A veterinary surgeon's experience when visiting their doctor...

Doctor's Appointment

I had a small taste of our local general practice this morning; a rather surreal experience.

It began with making the appointment last week, in no rush. I called the practice number in the directory and was given a series of telephone options and when I took the fifth one for appointments, an answer machine message gave me another (not listed in the directory) telephone number.

Having met an engaged tone most of the morning, I eventually got through to a human: when I asked for an appointment I was told '...well, the earliest 'bookable' appointment will be next Wednesday....' This is all a bit weird because I was also told that I could have had an appointment within 48 hours at an 'appointed' time, it's just that it wouldn't have been a 'bookable' appointment. Actually, I don't care whether I have a 'bookable' as opposed to any other appointment...

On the allotted day, I arrived and stood behind the person who was using the automatic booking in machine. It wasn't working, so I went straight up to the reception – six feet away – and announced myself. The receptionist asked if I had booked in automatically. I said no, because the machine wasn't working. She then said, 'Well, really you should use the automated booking-in machine'. I asked her to make an exception – please – because the machine was broken. 'Oh it's broken again is it?' she replied. This scene repeated throughout my stay as more and more people told her. She told them all they should have used the machine.

I was directed to sit 'over there' and joined ten others sitting in rows in a waiting room with no dog-eared magazines of any description. Instead, the walls had wall charts of severe information on Alzheimer's and Dementia and Diabetes – nothing on Pet Smiles or Fat Dogs or Fleas with fangs, so perhaps we are out of step in actually being humorous about disease.

All the others waiting clearly had neck problems because they were all sitting gazing fixedly upward at a mesmeric series of messages on an electronic screen. Some people had been there so long they even had 'O' sign with a faint trail of dribble on their cheek depending on whether their heads inclined to the left or right.

The messages varied from: 'Speak to the receptionist if your appointment is twenty minutes over'. Given the observed behaviour of the receptionist, I didn't hold out much hope of anything other than being told to use the machine again.

To BEEEEEEEEEEEEEPPP! (the sign made a severe noise) 'Mr. Smith to see Dr Newman'. This caused a spasm each time in those in the waiting room and handkerchiefs or shirt sleeves wiped away the gobs. God, people are attractive.

(Continued)

Box 4.1   Cont'd

I fell asleep as my waiting time went well over half an hour and a kindly client – also waiting – nudged me when it was my turn.

The GP didn't get out of her chair to examine me and pronounced my mole a mole or rather 99.9% likely to be a mole. That's better, I hope...!

I went to work, found my smiling receptionists laughing with clients, taking telephone calls with enthusiasm and asking how it went – in front of a full waiting room.... So I told them.

And then next week I have the dentist...

ANON

YOUR PROFESSIONAL PERSONALITY

Your professional personality must be appropriate to:

- you – so that you can be natural
- your practice – as a representative of it!
- your client – they are individuals.

Now consider the exercise in figure 4.1.

Figure 4.1   Exercise: Responding to a forced smile

Imagine yourself in any situation where you have been greeted with a forced smile. This could be in a store, in a restaurant, in a wine bar or perhaps in a bank or building society! What were your reactions? What do you think the forced smile communicated? Jot down some of the words that spring to mind as you imagine yourself back in the situation.

-
-
-
-
-

Words which may have appeared on your list might include:

- insincerity
- superficiality
- untrustworthiness
- plastic, false, fake
- patronizing
- off-putting.

So, obviously, this 'false smile' approach to welcoming clients does not work. How about the opposite of this, when someone serving you is rude or indifferent? You probably come away feeling dissatisfied or just angry.

As a professional person, you need to find a middle course through these two kinds of service so that you and your clients feel comfortable and your practice is also comfortable and happy with your approach.

Nobody is asking you to change your whole personality or to pretend to be impossibly cheery all of the time. The main thing to remember is that however you choose to be welcoming should be appropriate to yourself. You might want to open up a conversation with a client, or you may prefer just to smile and say 'hello'.

However good you already are at this, there is still room for improvement. You will continue to learn as you practise your skills.

DEVELOPING RELATIONSHIPS AND BUILDING RAPPORT

As a representative of your veterinary practice, you need to maintain a professional attitude to your job. It's up to you to make clients feel welcome.

The skills involved in building ordinary relationships and establishing contact and rapport with clients are basically the same. You need to be comfortable using these skills in order to do your job well.

THE ART OF CLIENT SERVICE IS MAKING PEOPLE FEEL SPECIAL

Making people feel special is one of the essential elements in forming relationships.

You can show that you think someone is worth your time and attention in many ways. It is this ability to show that you feel this – and not just say it – that makes good relationships. This is true of any relationship, whether it is an intimate partnership or a professional contact with a client. Like so many other personal skills, this can be learned and developed.

The quiz (Figure 4.2) asks you to assess your attitude to relationships in general. That attitude is central to your attitude to client service.

In a client service situation, you have just ten seconds to start building a relationship with your client.

How did you do?

If your total score was between 45 and 50, your attitude to people you come into contact with is a positive, open one. The relationship you build with clients is likely to be successful. However, there is always a risk you might have an off day and someone will not see you quite as you'd like.

If you scored 35–44, your attitude tends to be more positive than negative, but you may find it hard to make initial contact. You will need to take note of the information in this section and polish-up that skill.

If you scored 25–34, you are not open to making new relationships and establishing contact with clients. You could do with being more open and tolerant. Providing good client care is a skill that can be developed if you are prepared to work at it – the pay-back to you is worth it.

Figure 4.2 Quiz: How positive is your attitude to relationships?

Put a tick in the appropriate column to indicate your level of agreement with each of the statements below to find out how positive your approach to other people is. Think about each one and answer honestly.

	Strongly Disagree	Disagree	Neither agree nor disagree	Agree	Strongly agree
Column score:	1	2	3	4	5
a) I like to spend time with other people					
b) Every human being is worthy of respect					
c) Every relationship involves give and take					
d) I am not afraid to talk openly about myself					
e) I am happy to hear what other people think about me and to tell them what I think about them					
f) I am willing to give help to other people and to ask for it when I need to					
g) Each individual is made up of a mixture of strengths and weaknesses					
h) I think most people respond positively if they are approached positively					
i) I don't expect to like everyone, or everyone to like me					
j) I can accept that other people don't always behave or turn out to be the way I want them to					
Score: (multiply the total number of ticks in each column by the column score)					
Sum all column scores to give you your Total Score:					

If you scored less than 25, your attitude tends to be more negative than positive, which makes it difficult for you to relax into a relationship or rapport. You could do with loosening up and practising the skills outlined in this section. Don't forget, some of your best friends were once strangers to you!

Remember: it is not enough to feel positive about your client; you must show it in your words and actions.

People cannot read your mind; they can only see your actions and hear your words.

Using the information from the previous exercise, write what you think you could make more of (your strengths) and what you could use less of (your weaknesses) in the spaces below:

I will do more of this:

■
■
■
■
■

I will do less of this:

■
■
■
■

> **SECTION SUMMARY**
> In this section, you have put yourself in the client's shoes to see how you respond to forced 'client service skills'. You have also explored your attitude to relationships in general and seen how building rapport with your client uses the same basic skills. You have assessed yourself on these and started to look at how you can improve. The next section gives you more information on how you can go about it.

THE GOLDEN RULES FOR MAKING PEOPLE FEEL SPECIAL

Research on the skills of building rapport and forming relationships shows clearly that people are attracted to other people who:

■ Have a positive attitude to themselves and other people.
■ Demonstrate energy and enthusiasm – they look as if they're glad to be there and have something to offer.
■ Make them feel special.

In this section, you will be looking at general rules to follow so that you can make your clients feel special.

You can do this by:

Being	Showing	Being	Showing	Building
T	R	U	S	T
R	E	N	E	
U	S	D	N	R
T	P	E	S	
H	E	R	I	U
F	C	S	T	
U	T	T	I	S
L		A	V	
		N	I	T
		D	T	
		I	Y	
		N		
		G		

The aim when working in veterinary practice is to build TRUST – that may be a client's trust in the veterinary surgeon's clinical diagnosis, to trust that they will not be over charged or sold something they did not need.

When clients visit your practice with their animals, what do they want? In broad terms, they want one of two things. They either have a healthy animal and want it to stay that way, because they have come in for a booster vaccination, or they perceive that their animal is unhealthy and want you to put matters right. Either way, they *trust* you with their animal's health and welfare. So, trust becomes the watchword for giving clients the confidence they need to bring their animals to you. And without animals being brought into your practice by their owners, you cannot offer the animal any care – and you have no job!

So, let us look at the components of trust in turn.

BE *TRUTHFUL* AND BE YOURSELF

Have you ever tried on an item of clothing and been uncertain about whether it suits you? The shop assistant may have urged you to buy the item and reassured you that it was right for you. Perhaps you took the advice and bought it, took it home only to find that your gut-reaction was reinforced by the comments of family or friends. Thinking back, you realized that the assistant was so keen to make the sale that he or she told you a 'white lie' to persuade you to buy. You probably wouldn't ever trust the assistant again. You might never return to the shop.

It is often tempting to tell people what you think they want to hear, rather than the truth. Doing this can get you into trouble and, in the end, it can make people learn to distrust your views.

It is a good rule to try to tell your clients the truth. By being truthful and being true to yourself.

However, in veterinary practice, there are times when you cannot be wholly truthful. The truth: 'your pet will die', or 'the vet does not want to talk to you and while he is here he has just asked me to tell you that he is not' might not be the best approach!

SHOW RESPECT

Showing respect for your clients: making them feel that they are important, is the first vital quality that helps to make them feel special. Try the quiz in figure 4.3.

Before moving on, let us consider some of the issues raised. What do you think of, for example, the first point – use a person's name? What do you do to remember that Mrs Jones wants to be called by her first name and finds 'Mrs' too formal, while Mrs Smyth does not like the informality of first name terms? How do you share this information so that your colleagues do not make the same mistake?

Number 7 may make you question the sense of the checklist. But remember, clients are pet owners so give them psychological 'stroking' and tell them something positive about their pet or the way they look after them.

Number 10 is so easy to get wrong without realizing it. When someone else makes a mistake: 'I am sorry, she is new here' (i.e. untrained) or when a client comes from the consulting room with a tube of a new ointment and asks what they are supposed to do with it: 'I am sorry, he's Belgian' (i.e. unclear) will not do! (The authors, while researching this book, witnessed both these responses!)

Figure 4.3   Quiz: How do you score on a dozen things to show respect to others?

Here is a list of a dozen smart things you can do to make clients feel important or show them respect. Tick the things that you do already: Do you....	
1. Use a person's name?	☐
2. Ask them questions to find out what they want?	☐
3. Show consideration?	☐
4. Show concern?	☐
5. Look at them when they are speaking?	☐
6. Ask their opinion?	☐
7. Tell them something you like about them?	☐
8. Remember something about them?	☐
9. Maintain politeness beyond the first contact?	☐
10. Not criticize clients or colleagues behind their back?	☐
11. Listen to them?	☐
12. Pay attention to them when they are waiting, responding if they become visibly agitated?	☐

SHOW YOUR CLIENTS THAT YOU UNDERSTAND

The second essential element in dealing with clients is the ability to see their point of view – to imagine what it is like to be them. (This was looked at in detail above.)

When you are serving a client, you need to recognize that they may have a different view of what is going on. You need to be able to put yourself in their place and anticipate their needs. Understanding, like respect, is a quality that not only has to be felt: you have to *show* it. If you can remember how it feels to be a client yourself, you will automatically be better at giving excellent service to your own clients.

When a client comes in with their cat that has an abscess on its jaw, how big is that abscess? Huge! How does it compare with the largest you have ever seen or how does it compare with the road traffic accident last week? Whatever your opinion, you must show your clients that you understand how they feel.

Can you think of ways that you can show your clients that you understand their point of view? Jot ideas down in the margin and then see if any of the suggestions matches yours.

> How can you show that you understand?
>
> Sensitivity – you pick up on how they feel as well as what they say and act accordingly.
>
> Expression – you show in your face that you are on the same wavelength; you look concerned if they are, amused if they are, and you respond.
>
> Values – you don't tell them what you think but accept what they say and listen carefully; what are their values?
>
> Empathize – you tell them about similar experiences that you have had or heard of.
>
> Sympathize – you show sympathy if necessary.

Showing that you are listening goes a long way towards making your clients feel that you understand them. This is not the passive process it seems to be at first. There are skills involved, and using these skills makes the difference between being a good listener and being a poor listener. (This reinforces what we said in Chapter 3.)

So what should we do – and not do – when speaking with clients? Go through the checklist in Figure 4.4, ticking the particular things you do while you are listening to somebody talking to you. Recognize and act on the don'ts as well as the do's.

We will explore your listening skills a little more in Chapter 8.

WINNING AND BUILDING THE CLIENT'S TRUST

Trust is the result of all of the other elements. Clients must feel that they can trust you and your practice. A false smile makes people feel uneasy. A client faced with this kind of welcome would feel uncomfortable. There would be no feeling of trust because the smile and the words do not seem to be genuine.

Figure 4.4 Quiz: How do you score on these do's and don'ts when listening to people?

Here is a list of five smart things you can do to help clients feel that you are genuinely listening to them – and five dumb things not to do! *Do you....*	
1. Look at the person who is speaking to you. Recognize how the speaker feels about what he or she is saying?	☺
2. Look for points to agree with rather than to argue with?	☺
3. Give a quick summary of what you have heard every now and again to check that it is correct?	☺

4. Give your full attention to the person who is speaking by
  ■ facing them
  ■ nodding your head
  ■ commenting to show you are still listening?
	☺

5. Take on board what is being said and not let prejudices get in the way?	☺
And you don't....	
6. Become negative about, or belittle, what the person is saying?	☹
7. Change the subject inappropriately?	☹
8. Fidget or distract the speaker?	☹
9. Let your eyes wander round the room?	☹
10. Criticize clients or colleagues in front of others in reception?	☹

Have a look at the quiz in Figure 4.5 to gauge how trustworthy you seem to be?

Figure 4.5 Quiz: How trustworthy do you appear to clients?

Here is a list of ways in which you can show that you are trustworthy. Do you do these things? *Tick the ones you do.*	
You are open and honest about yourself and the practice. (Don't say you can do something if you can't)	☐
You admit your mistakes if you have made them. (Always apologize on behalf of the practice even if it's not your fault) Important: See p 103	☐
You keep your promises. (Make sure you can!)	☐
You follow your promises up with actions. (See that this is done – check it out)	☐
You respect confidences. (Don't gossip about clients)	☐
You put yourself out to help other people. (Always be willing and helpful)	☐
You are what you seem to be. (If you can do all this, you will be!)	☐

SECTION SUMMARY
The essential elements for establishing contact and making relationships with clients are:

- being truthful
- showing respect
- being understanding
- showing sensitivity.

These all add up to:

- winning and building TRUST.

As your clients can only judge you on what they can see and hear, you have to make an effort to demonstrate these qualities. You can succeed by remembering the circumstances and tips described in this section.

RESPONDING TO INDIVIDUAL CLIENTS AND MATCHING THEIR NEEDS

Different clients have different needs. Your approach to client service also has to be appropriate to the needs of your individual clients. As said, all people need a certain degree of care and respect, but treating everyone exactly the same ignores individual needs. Considering all that you have learnt so far, what do you think the particular needs of the kinds of people in Figure 4.6 might be? Make a note of the things you would do and those you would not do in the spaces below each brief description of a type of client. The first example has been done to give you the idea.

DEALING WITH SPECIAL NEEDS CLIENTS

There will be situations where you may have to deal with people who have 'special needs'. Try not to make any assumptions about the intelligence, personality or interests of anyone with impairment. Think positively about what they can do rather than what they cannot do.

Clients with hearing impairments

It is said that one in six people has some form of hearing problems – and it is not solely the preserve of the elderly. Sadly, being deaf seems to be the hub of many music hall jokes, yet the condition – often linked with tinnitus (a severe ringing in the ears) – is anything but funny. The author's late mother was profoundly deaf since the Second World War; she said that, if anything, she'd much prefer to be deaf than blind (being deaf was easier than being blind); however, it did not have the same visible signs of impairment and left many thinking that she was either rude or stupid (when she was far from either!).

Do remember, that while people may not have any visible signs of deafness (and many people do not admit that they have a problem), be patient with others before

Figure 4.6   How might you treat these different types of clients so they feel as individuals?

1. A shy person
Do *Explain things clearly, ask questions, be patient and put them at their ease. Smile, talk softly.*
Don't *Treat them as a nuisance. Rush them or make them speak up in front of a full waiting room.*
2. An elderly person who is a little confused
Do
Don't
3. A scruffy or badly dressed person
Do
Don't
4. A well-dressed, well-groomed person
Do
Don't
5. A very talkative person
Do
Don't
6. Someone who does not speak English very well or who has difficulty in expressing themselves
Do
Don't
7. A positive, friendly person
Do
Don't
8. A negative, grumpy person
Do
Don't
9. An impatient person
Do
Don't
10. A demanding, angry person
Do
Don't

jumping to any conclusions. If you feel that the other person has some hearing impairment, there are a number of things that you can do to help people.

- Turn your face so it is fully visible when you speak
- If possible, use the client's name
- Speak normally – slow your rate of speaking very slightly
- Don't distort your normal lip patterns or natural rhythm
- Don't shout – it is painful for the client. It also distorts your lips and face, which interferes with the client's reading ability
- Make sure nothing is in the way or that anything at all is obstructing any part of your face. For example, your hand on or over your face, pen in your mouth or chewing gum. Be aware that beards and moustaches could be a problem – they cause an obstruction making lip reading difficult, or impossible
- Don't be put off by voices that sound strange. Profoundly deaf clients cannot hear the sounds they are making and may mispronounce unfamiliar words
- If the hearing-impaired person has a sign language interpreter with them, talk to the client, not the interpreter, i.e. make sure you are facing the client and follow all the other guidelines here
- If you need to attract the attention of someone with hearing problems touch them lightly on their shoulder or upper arm – do not grab them or touch them anywhere else

Conversing

When speaking to a client with hearing impairments:

- Try to be in a well-lit area
- Always have the light in your face
- Minimize noise as far as possible as hearing-impaired clients are unable to be selective as to what they pick up. A hearing aid amplifies everything. For example, if you are in a noisy office and there are other conversations going on, the aid will amplify them all and your client may be unable to distinguish between conversations.

If you have trouble in communicating, write it down. It doesn't give offence. Many people with hearing impairments carry notebooks.

Lastly, and most importantly, treat all people with hearing impairments as people!

CLIENTS WITH VISUAL IMPAIRMENTS

Many people seem to assume that a visually impaired person is also hearing impaired. This usually isn't so, and the opposite may well be true – their hearing may have become particularly acute as compensation – so resist any temptation to shout.

Clients with visual impairments may sometimes appear offhand. They are not – they may not react in the way you expect because they have only one dimension to work on, as they are unable to read body language. From bitter experience they may also be fiercely independent and not appreciate assistance when they are manoeuvring through the doors. While it is a natural reaction to welcome a client's animal and make a fuss of it – guide dogs should be left alone: they are working!

Conversing

If the client is partially sighted, be very clear in your body language – using verbal signs and clear gestures.

When giving directions, be specific. For example: Do not say: 'the seats are over there', but: 'if you turn around, the seats will be on your right, approximately 3 yards forwards and one yard to your right'.

Your practice can assist by having Braille or large type for specific instructions when written material is needed. Large type should be produced on A4 paper; not just A4 enlarged to A3, which is unwieldy.

If the client with visual impairments has a human guide – as with the hearing impaired guide – do not speak to them instead of the client.

Treat the client as a person.

CLIENTS WITH SPEECH IMPAIRMENTS

While perhaps less common than hearing and sight impairments, speech impairments include:

- indistinct speech
- stammering
- an inability to speak.

Conversing

Do not finish sentences for clients: no matter how tempting and no matter how quickly you think it will move the conversation on.

Be very careful about your body language – it is very easy to signal negatively to a client without saying a word.

If your client's impairment is severe, then it is likely that they will not be offended if you ask them to write something down. They are also likely to carry a notebook. For example: 'I am sorry, I couldn't quite understand that. Would you write it down for me?'

Clients with speech impairments are usually able bodied in every other way.

Treat them as people.

Suggested answers for 'matching the clients' needs' exercise in Figure 4.6

2. An elderly person who is a little confused

Do: *Elderly people generally appreciate a friendly smile. Show that you recognize them, if you do. Show an interest in them and make conversation. They appreciate a little of your time.*

Don't: *Be patronizing and talk to them like babies – or be impatient and intolerant. Don't make fun if they are hard of hearing.*

3. A scruffy or badly dressed person

Do: *This person deserves as much respect and courtesy as anyone. They may need a welcome and be put at ease.*

Don't: *Dismiss them as if they do not matter. Appearances can lie, and this person could want to buy up the whole practice – you could have put them off! And don't assume they have no money to pay the bill.*

4. A well-dressed, well-groomed person

Do: *People who are well-turned-out have put a lot of effort into their overall presentation. They often expect to be treated with respect and appreciation. A good, professional approach should satisfy everyone, not just the well-groomed.*

Don't: *Grovel or be off-hand. Don't give them extended credit without authority and don't assume that they will pay the bill either!*

5. A very talkative person

Do: *Listen carefully. They can be confusing, so try to sort out exactly what it is they want. Repeat what you think they want to be sure you have it right. Keep them to the point.*

Don't: *Butt in and anticipate what they are going to say before you are sure of what it is, and don't be drawn into a conversation about something else.*

6. Someone who does not speak English well, or who has difficulty in expressing themselves

Do: *Listen carefully and watch their gestures. Explain things simply and clearly, using gestures and pointing.*

Don't: *Show impatience, or interrupt too soon.*

7. A positive, friendly person

Do: *Respond cheerfully and positively. Make the most of this person.*

Don't: *Take this person for granted, and treat them casually because they won't make a fuss.*

8. A negative, grumpy person

Do: *Be sympathetic but cheerful. Show them you understand and are willing to help. Be professional.*

Don't: *Take their attitude personally and be pulled into a negative frame of mind yourself. It's not you they are grumpy about, it's probably the world!*

9. An impatient person

Do: *Be as efficient as you can. Apologize politely. Explain why there may have been a delay, and tell them what is happening. Explain how much longer you are likely to be.*

Don't: *Allow yourself to be hurried into making mistakes or becoming flustered.*

10. A demanding, angry person

Do: *Be polite and patient. Show that you are listening carefully to them and that you understand. Keep calm, and above all: be professional.*

Don't: *Be drawn into an argument, and don't take their anger personally.*

SECTION SUMMARY

Different clients have different needs. The skill of really good client care is in identifying these needs and being flexible and sensitive enough to meet them. All clients need to feel cared for and special – they also need to feel that you are treating them as an individual, not just another client.

KEYTIPS: MAKING THE CLIENT FEEL SPECIAL

1. They need to feel *welcome* (respect, understanding).
2. They need to feel *comfortable* (understanding).
3. They need to be *understood* (understanding).
4. They need *assistance* (understanding).
5. They need to feel *important* (respect).
6. They need to be *recognized* (respect).
7. They need to be treated with *respect* (respect).
8. They need to be *listened to* (understanding).
9. They need prompt *service* (respect).
10. They need to *trust* you (trust).

CHECKLIST (PIN UP IN YOUR KITCHEN!)

- Be welcoming to your client.
- Show your client that they count.
- Respect your employer.
- Respond to the client's individual needs.
- Have a positive attitude.
- Demonstrate energy and enthusiasm.
- Make your client feel special.
- Develop trust.
- Tell your client the truth.
- Show your client that you respect them.
- Ask them questions.
- Be polite.
- Use their name.
- Listen to the client.
- Show your client that you understand.
- Be sensitive to your client's needs.
- Admit mistakes when you have made them.
- Keep your promises.
- Respect confidences.
- Be yourself.

Chapter 5

Telephone skills

BT maintains that 98% of clients' initial contact with the practice is by phone. This is why good telephone skills are essential. No matter how good the practice is, the way that first phone call is handled is crucial to the old or new client coming to the practice with their pet. For many new clients the phone is the *first* contact with the practice. It's important that it is not the last. This call can win or lose clients.

You represent the practice. You have to rely on your voice and telephone manner to sell the practice. You should regard the telephone as a friend rather than a foe, although it has a nasty habit of ringing when you are busy dealing with clients at reception. Like it or not, it is your contact with the outside world.

For old or new clients, this point of contact is the major source of business for your practice. The practice needs this work to stay in business. It keeps you in a job.

Yes, *that's* how important your telephone skills are – they help keep *you* in a job!

Perhaps the best way to understand how important it is, comes from taking note of what other organizations sound like when you contact them. Doctors, hairdressers, laboratories, DEFRA, drug companies, shops, take-aways, listen carefully to them all and review them critically in your own mind. Would you like to sound like them? Why? What was good about it and what left you wondering?

So what are the skills you need?

The next step is to try to assess how *you* sound on the phone. Would you like to be treated that way? Are you falling into habits that you don't like in other organizations?

Try to develop a style of your own that includes all the good points of other people and avoids all the mistakes. There is no need to conform to a strict pattern if you have your own style that works well.

All that has been said about first impressions in Chapter 2 applies to this telephone contact, but what a disadvantage you are at – the caller can't see you. You have got to get all the right messages across to the caller using only your voice. You can't establish any eye contact, you can't see how they are reacting to you. People listen more acutely on the telephone because the ear is the only point of contact. They are more easily distracted by background noises so they need to be kept to a minimum. Do they see what they hear?

Whether your job involves staying in one position to use the phone, as a receptionist might, for example, or answering any phone, anywhere in the building, all the points in this chapter are important.

PREPARATION FOR INCOMING CALLS

Place – where is the phone? Is it accessible? Which hand is easier for you to talk and write with?

Recognizing clients – regular clients expect it, but it is not an easy skill.

Recording information – always have a pen and paper handy. A messages book is far better than scraps of paper which are easily lost.

Know the whereabouts of people – if you don't know, don't admit it! Say they are in theatre and will call you back. *You* make sure they do. You promised.

Making contact – get the message through, too. If you are going to contact someone, say you are going to call them on their mobile rather than 'I'll see if they are around'.

Practice policy – what do you do about transferring calls, quoting prices; availability of vets should be known beforehand, not during a call.

More than one call – it will depend on the phone system you have as to what you can do. Know what the policy is and who will pick up the next call.

PRACTICE PHONE POLICY

Does the practice have a phone answering policy? If not, here are some ideas, to consider in creating a policy.

Practice phone policy should address the following:

- How long do you allow the phone to ring before answering it?
- Do staff have a script for answering the phone, not perhaps a good idea, scripts tend to sound false and patronizing?
- Who needs to be taken care of first, the waiting room client or the phone caller?
- Have you been trained in how to answer the phone?
- How do you handle the phone shopper?
- Do you have Call Minder™ or a call waiting system?
- Do you smile when you answer the phone?

SOMEBODY ANSWER THAT PHONE!

Three rings is the norm, answer any sooner than three and the caller will not have had time to compose themselves as to what they want to say to you. Three rings on your phone, equates to only two at the caller's end. Answering the phone on one ring implies that you are not busy and hovering over it waiting for it to ring.

LET ME SEE THE SCRIPT

Everyone, and that includes the veterinary surgeons, who is likely to answer the phone should all use a similar greeting but not so that it becomes stereotyped. Not just 'Hello', which usually gets the caller response of 'Is that the Vets?'. Try not to make the greeting sound too much like you are reading from a script, and don't make it so long that it has cost the caller 20p before they have told you what they want. A simple greeting, the name of the practice, and how can you help will suffice. Whether you include your name is up to you, remember personal security.

Many service company's phone greetings are obviously scripted and sound false and insincere. They generate the totally wrong impression, which is the last thing you want to do.

ALWAYS TRY TO CONVEY THE BEST POSSIBLE IMAGE TO THE CALLER

Don't say: 'Who's calling', this always sounds very abrupt and offhand.
Say: 'May I ask who's calling?'
Don't say: 'He hasn't come in yet', this implies he's late for work.
Say: 'He's not in the practice at the moment.'
Don't say: 'He's gone home early', again this sounds like the person has skipped off early.
Say: 'He'll be back in the practice tomorrow morning at…'
Never say: 'He/she is at the hairdressers!'

TAKE CARE OF THE CLIENT IN FRONT OF YOU FIRST

If you are dealing with a client in the waiting room when the phone goes, by allowing it to ring three times, you have the opportunity to apologize to the client for the interruption. Ask them if they mind you taking the call. Then answer the phone (see the seven Ps on p. 67). It also allows you to get paper and pen ready to take a message.

TRAINING ON HOW TO ANSWER THE PHONE

All practices should spend time on training staff how to answer the phone correctly. Being told, 'there's the phone' is not good enough. Neither should training be just a 'one off' when staff join the practice, but reviewed on a regular basis.

'Could you tell me how much…?' Every day you will get callers wanting to know how much your fees are for a particular procedure. Handling these calls correctly can generate new business. Before giving the information required, ask some questions about the pet – its age, breed and sex. Also ask them for an address so you can send them a copy of the practice brochure (if you have one). Then tell them what they want to know and explain why your practice offers the best in petcare. Show an interest in their situation, and try to provide solutions.

'THE OTHER PERSON KNOWS YOU ARE WAITING'...ARRGH!

Phone companies go to great lengths to sell us call monitoring systems, like *Call Minder* or *Call Waiting*™. If you have ever been on the receiving end of *Call Waiting*™ – then beware! This system in the authors' opinion is *not* for veterinary practice. Not only do you get an annoying bleep during the conversation you are engaged in, but the caller keeps getting the message that you know there is another call coming in. How do they then feel when the message tells them to call back later? Great, if you are the client with an animal that has been involved in an RTA. Far better to be met by an engaged signal.

    Call Minder™, however, acts like an answering machine, while you are on the line and invites the caller to leave a short message, so you can call them back when you are free. You can, if required, tailor the message on the system to your practice. Also, this system will actually phone you to remind you that you have messages to attend to, should you forget to check periodically.

AUTOMATED HANDLING SYSTEMS

These are the systems that take you through an extensive menu of services – 'If you have a touch tone, press star; if you need accounts, press 1', etc.– and may work well for very large organizations, but not for a practice. Figure 5.1 sums up our feelings of automation. Again imagine the client with their pet that has just been involved in an accident, they don't want to know you have an accounts department or a grooming service, they want to speak to a vet. This system falls into the same category as *Call Waiting*™.

Figure 5.1   Don't let your clients lose the will to live!

CAN THEY HEAR YOU SMILE?

It is very easy to detect a smile over the phone, because smiling involves changes in the facial muscles and, as a consequence, the voice changes, and the caller will get the impression that you are smiling, which in turn generates a feeling of warmth and well being.

OTHER CONSIDERATIONS

Other areas to consider are:

- Tone of voice – speak clearly and slowly, not too slowly so the caller feels like a half wit.
- Jargon – avoid jargon which may confuse the caller.
- Keep confidentiality, the waiting room may hear you; it's a captive audience!

USING THE TELEPHONE (MAKING CALLS)

Occasionally, you will be asked to phone the wholesaler, or some other organization, with a query. All the points about voice and demeanour are equally important for the outgoing call. There are one or two other things worth considering, since you can exercise more control because you are choosing to make the call. They won't avoid all frustrations, but they will help.

PREPARATION

Timing

Very often there is no option but to make a call without being able to plan the timing. However, calls that can be planned are more efficient and quicker. The telephone bill is one way in which organizations can make considerable savings by using a bit of discipline and that's where you can help. Even if the rates are lowered, keep it simple. Overseas calls should be planned to coincide with waking hours in the other country.

Telephone numbers

Make sure you have the right number. Don't trust your memory, except for the most frequently made calls. Wrong numbers cost money and are frustrating. Use a directory. Make a practice directory of your most useful numbers and keep it by the phone. Use it to keep a note of numbers that you have had difficulty finding. Use your system's stored numbers facility if it has one, to avoid mistakes in dialling:

- DEFRA
- Taxis
- Veterinary Investigation Centres (VICs)
- Diagnostic labs
- Pharmaceutical companies technical services
- Crematoria
- Abattoirs

Extension numbers

Always use an extension number if you know it. Ask the receptionist for the number rather than the person. Many organizations now have the facility to dial an extension direct, without going through an exchange receptionist. It all saves time, and that means money, as usual.

Reason for call

Have a clear reason for calling, and stick to it. Maybe jot down the reason on a piece of paper.

DOCUMENTS

When you are making the call, there can be no excuse for not having the appropriate documents to hand. 'Hang on while I just check my records' is not very impressive when you knew what you might need before making the call. Don't feel annoyed with yourself if you do feel some anxiety. It is perfectly natural and a moderate level of nerves can actually add to your performance as the adrenaline brings an extra sharpness to your mind.

DIFFICULT CALLS

When making a call where you want to be assertive, maybe you are complaining about the high number of 'to follow' items from your wholesaler, make the call standing up, and visualize the person at the other end sitting down. The psychology of this situation is quite powerful.

Here is a simple but highly effective six point plan to see you through those calls you would rather avoid making. It takes a moment but gets results.

Six point plan

1. Decide on a specific time – about 15 minutes in the future – when you will pick up the phone and dial the number. If you've got a watch with an alarm, set it. It is important, though, to pick a time when the person will be able to take the call.
2. While waiting, plan what you want to say. It often helps to jot down the key points.
3. Relax briefly by sitting down and closing your eyes. Focus on your breathing and, each time you exhale, feel yourself becoming calmer. It deepens the relaxation to repeat the phrase 'calm and relaxed' with each exhaled breath.
4. Imagine yourself making the call confidently and calmly. See yourself putting across all the salient points in a clear, assertive manner and dealing with any objections that arise with the same assurance.
5. As soon as the time for making the call arrives, pick up the phone and dial without further hesitation.

6. After the call, reflect on how it went. Pick out all the positive aspects of your performance and congratulate yourself on them. Next consider anything interesting which happened, whether or not it was positive. Only after this should you explore any negative aspects and think about how these might be changed and improved upon in the future.

PRESENTATION
Identification

Never assume you are connected to the person you expected. If they don't immediately identify themselves, always check that you're speaking to the right person. There is nothing more frustrating than having to repeat yourself.

Introduction

Introduce yourself clearly and precisely and say what practice you are calling from. Quickly establish the subject of your call.

Records

Keep permanent notes of the relevant details of the conversation.

PROBLEMS
Holding on

If you are asked to hold on while someone is found, or a document is looked for, try to get some idea of the time it will take. If there is likely to be a substantial delay, ask if you could be called back, and give your number, even if the person already has it. Alternatively, say you will call back at a pre-arranged time, and establish what the best time will be.

Calling back

If you have been promised a call back, at a certain time, and it doesn't happen, call again 15 minutes after the appointed time, and ask politely to speak with the person again. If they have not had the message, or have failed to respond to it, and are not available again, explain clearly what has happened, in somewhat icier tones than normal, but remain polite. Usually, it will not be the message carrier's fault, but they will be more anxious to help you to make the contact if you remain reasonable.

Leaving messages

Tread carefully. It may be more appropriate to leave a message rather than call again, but not necessarily. If it is, make sure the message is clear and concise, and if it involves dates, times or telephone numbers, or other confusable details don't be afraid to ask the message carrier to repeat them back to you to check. Quite often numbers are written down wrongly, even with the best intentions. Ask a dozen people to write down 90996, and unless you prepare them, at least one of them is likely to write 90966, or 90096. Try it. When leaving messages on voice mail, always repeat your phone number.

Disconnection

If you have made the call and are cut off, put the phone down and dial again immediately. Don't wait for the other party to reconnect – you are the one that definitely knows the number without having to wait to look it up. Get in quickly before another call engages the line.

UNWANTED CALLS

We hope this never happens. Occasionally, you will be at the receiving end of a malicious or obscene telephone call to the surgery. The golden rule is not to get involved in a dialogue with the caller. That's just what they want you to do. In such situations, the answer is simple – *hang up*. Older members of staff may think it's a joke, but to younger members that call may be particularly distressing. If the problem persists then you should contact BT and ask them to monitor your line.

You may also be at the receiving end of a tirade of verbal abuse from a client. Again, you are not paid to be subject to abuse. With this type of call you should say, 'I am afraid I do not have to listen to such language, I am now terminating this call', and hang up. If you are not sure who the client was, dial 1471 to find out. Do not swear back, however tempting, it might cost you your job. *Now, it is extremely important that your employers have a very strong policy on these calls.* There have been cases where clients who have been abusive on the phone to staff phone the practice Principal to complain about the receptionist's attitude!

FAX MESSAGES

Fax machines can offer tremendous improvements to communications, but they have their limitations, and there are a few points to remember:

FAX NUMBERS

Always check the number and re-check it when you have entered it. It may be very important that the fax goes only to the right person. If you rely on the machine's stored numbers with abbreviated dialling, it is even more important that you check that you have the code right, before you send.

INFORMATION/ACTION

If you are merely passing on information, it may not be important that the fax is not read straight away. Because you cannot be sure that anyone will receive it at the time you send it, messages that require action are better passed by phone, or phone and fax.

CONFIDENTIALITY

Basically, there is no confidentiality in sending faxes. If you wish to attempt to restrict the number of people who can read your fax, you must telephone first, speak to the person for whom the message is intended, and ask them to stand by their fax machine. If you wish to check that it has arrived safely, ask them to phone or fax back to say they have received it.

CLARITY

Lab results: are they legible? – Phone to check.

THE DON'T LIST

Copy this list out and put it by the phone; it applies to *everyone* in the practice.

- DON'T have a three-way conversation.
- DON'T munch your snack or lunch in the mouthpiece.
- DON'T cover the phone – use the mute button.
- DON'T swear back.
- DON'T be too familiar.
- DON'T talk too long.

Three-way conversations are hard for you to follow and confuse the client and the other person involved because no one really knows who's talking to whom.

Eating when answering the phone is very rude and, because of the amplification on modern handsets, the noise is deafening to the caller. The best rule is not to eat when in the reception area, save the digestive biscuits until it is breaktime.

Not only do modern handsets amplify sounds, they are very sensitive, and pick up sounds through the back of the set. It is not an effective way temporarily to cut off a caller. Use the mute button, so any derogatory remarks made to a colleague are not likely to be heard by the caller! When you do use the mute button *do* tell the caller what you are doing. There is nothing so unprofessional as to be met with a deafening wall of silence.

No one ever won an argument by swearing back. It is very unprofessional and will not help client–practice relationships. Don't forget the waiting room 'audience', they can only hear your side of the conversation.

Familiarity on the phone is unnecessary and embarrassing, especially to those in the waiting room who have to listen to your call.

Keep talk time to a minimum, hard at times with the aged client who likes to phone up for that 'chat'. Remember that the long call is blocking the main line to the practice and you may have a client with an emergency call trying to get through, and you cannot be dealing with other clients. There are times when it may be necessary to invent an excuse for closing a conversation rather than just putting the phone down. 'I am sorry I must go now someone has just brought an emergency in' (perhaps not a good one to try as everyone in the waiting room looks at you in disbelief) or 'there is a call coming in on our emergency line, I must go now'.

THE SEVEN 'P'S OF THE PHONE

- Promptness
- Politeness
- Preparation
- Precision
- Professionalism
- Practicality
- Positivism

Reflect on what each of the above words means for you and write a few notes on a note pad or add to the Appendix.

PROACTIVE USE OF THE PHONE

How often does the practice have 'no shows' for elective surgery? The cost to the practice in time and money can be considerable. Clients simply have forgotten that their pet was due at the vets for an operation that had been arranged several weeks before.

So how can using the phone avoid such a situation?

Look at the time this way, illustrated in figure 5.2:

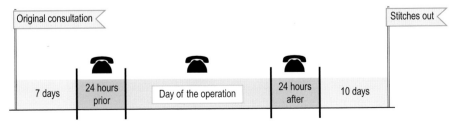

Figure 5.2 The time-line for a client around an operation

The original consultation, when it was decided that it would be in the best interests of the animal to have an operation, could be some time before the agreed date. Now the day before the operation is due, the practice phones the owner to remind them that they are looking forward to seeing their pet tomorrow. (Invariably met with, 'Oh, I had forgotten, thank you for reminding me'.) They remind them that the animal should not have anything to eat after a certain time, and water should be restricted and to walk the dog before coming in, to empty the bowels. It also provides an opportunity to answer any question the owners have.

On the day of 'the Op', the animal is admitted, the owners ask when they can phone to find out how everything has gone. Here is an opportunity for you to take control. Tell them you will phone when the operation has been done. Make sure that you have the number(s) where they can be contacted during the day. Tell them this for two reasons:

1. You don't know where the animal will be on the Op list; it will depend on an assessment of all the day's cases first.
2. You won't have all the owners whose pets are in that day phoning the practice at the same time and not being able to get through. The authors know of practices where the senior partner actually speaks on the phone from the theatre, to tell the owner how things have gone. This is client care *par excellence*. A proactive call also allows you to remind them that you will have their bill made out for their convenience and anything else they need can be easily added. (A subtle way of saying bring your cheque book or credit card.)

At discharge time tell the client that you will give them a call the following day.

This is not to advise them that you have lost a towel clip and would they watch the dog's stool for the next few days, but just to check everything is alright and there are no problems that are worrying them. Also it will give you another chance to remind them of the stitches out appointment, an appointment date that is often forgotten by the client in the exuberance of being reunited with their pet.

Many practices will baulk at the cost of making these calls, which should cost less than 20p each. But consider the goodwill they generate, definitely more than 20p.

ADD VALUE TO THAT CALL

Have all information to hand – surgery times, fees. A good idea is to keep all these in a folder at the reception desk.

GOOD LISTENING SKILLS

Respond appropriately (see Chapter 8).
Keep the phone separate from the rest of the reception area.

CALL MANAGEMENT

Which is the most important telephone line in your practice? In or Out? BT will run a usage check on your lines to monitor traffic. This will give you and the practice the opportunity to plan staffing of reception at peak phone times. One line ex-directory is good for out-going calls perhaps, or use the fax line when traffic is less.

Personal calls: what is the policy?

Calls to labs, wholesalers, discharge times, calls to other suppliers.

CHECKLIST

- Phone in a convenient place (if you have to have it in the reception area).
- Message book by the phone, with something to write with.
- Practice policy on abusive calls.
- Practice policy on how much information you can give out over the phone.
- List of useful numbers by the phone.

FURTHER INFORMATION

British Telecom: www.bt.com

Complaints about a phone service provider: www.ofcom.org.uk

Chapter 6

Professional under pressure

However good you are at dealing with clients and managing your 'moments of truth', however hard you try to make your clients feel special, there will be times when you are under pressure and it is difficult to keep smiling. You may be faced with an angry client or you may be rushed off your feet and still have to think about your clients' needs first.

This chapter focuses on how you can stay professional, keep cool and manage stressful situations. When you have reviewed it, you will be reminded how to do this and be professional under pressure.

Section 1 asks you to assess your overall level of stress at work and gives tips for minimizing it.

Section 2 looks at how to turn potentially negative situations into positive ones by 'positive self-talk'.

Section 3 is about dealing with difficult situations and how to keep smiling under attack.

Section 4 focuses on assertiveness – what it is and how to achieve it.

A NOTE FOR HEAD RECEPTIONISTS AND MANAGERS

In Mackay, 2007a, he concluded that, included under the heading of mental ill-health, too many people took time off for stress. Figures from a recent survey (Smith et al, 2000) provided an estimate of 13.4 million working days lost in Britain each year due to stress, depression or anxiety. This survey estimated that, on average, each sufferer took 29 days off work because of their complaint. This compares with 6.5 million working days lost and average days lost of 16 per affected person estimated from similar studies (Health and Safety Statistics Highlights 2001/02).

Calculations based on an HSE (Health and Safety Executive) report (HSE information sheet 2/99/EMSU) estimated that for work-related stress the cost to employers was about £353 million to £381 million (1995/96 prices) and to society about £3.7 to £3.8 billion. It should be noted that since these calculations were done, the estimated number of days lost due to stress has more than doubled.

HSE's key messages on stress are:

Work-related stress is a serious problem for organizations. Tackling it effectively can result in significant benefits for organizations.

There are things organizations can do to prevent and control work-related stress.

The law requires organizations to take action.

See also the International Stress Management Association at www.isma.org.uk and the Mental Health Foundation at www.mentalhealth.org.uk

STRESS – TOO MUCH, TOO LITTLE?

Are you over-stressed or just under too much pressure?

Coping with difficult situations and clients, and perhaps with other worries at work or at home, puts you under pressure. Too much of that pressure results in you being over-stressed. If you are, you will find it difficult to think positively and be professional.

This section looks at:

- Stress and your work
- The symptoms of over-stress and
- A few tips for minimizing your stress levels.

There is no maximum or minimum level of pressure that applies to everyone; each person has his or her own level. High pressure of one kind for one person may be fine for them, yet it may be too much for another. If you are not veterinary qualified you would probably consider that having to perform an ovarian hysterectomy on a Labrador would be too much pressure and would lead you to show symptoms of stress. Yet your veterinary surgeons develop the knowledge and skills to do this sort of operation calmly without undue pressure. However, some people *need* more pressure than others do. It is all down to the type of person we are.

Approximately 80% of all illness is stress-related.

Too much stress for you puts you into a possible 'danger zone' where you are more likely to become ill or to have an accident. Research shows that you are about 80% more accident-prone when over-stressed. You can also suffer from not having enough stress. The symptoms are similar to those of depression – tiredness and inability to face even the smallest tasks.

Read through the list of 'Stress Factors in Work' in Figure 6.1 and put a tick in the box beside any of the statements that apply to you or have applied to you in the last two months. To get a total score, add up the numbers beside each of your ticks. These are only 'clues' to your stress levels and are meant only as a guide. You may need more stress in your life than other people, for instance; or difficulties with your boss may rate as high for you as losing your job.

It is as well to remember those good things or changes in your life can be just as stressful as bad things are, although you may not feel them as such.

Stress can be defined based on perception:

Stress is the perceived demands of the situation balanced by the perceived ability of the person to deal with the situation.

Various chapters of this book are designed to help you improve your ability to cope with client interactions and to deal with the variety of situations that come your way working as a receptionist in veterinary practice.

To review the checklist for stress factors in work in Figure 6.1, if you have scored 20 or more, you are in the 'danger zone'. You should think hard about how you can cut down on the stress – or alternatively just wait. Some of the high scores may be because of a change in circumstances and the stress caused by this will decrease with time.

If you have scored 10–19 you should be thinking of ways to minimize stress in the areas of your life that you have control over.

Figure 6.1 Checklist: Stress factors at work

Stress factor	Relative stress	✓
You've started work for the first time or you've returned after a long absence.	2	
You are constantly overworked.	4	
You have to deal with difficult client complaints or emergencies most of the time.	3	
You have a major anxiety at work (the threat of losing your job, for instance).	4	
You are changing or have changed your job.	3	
You have been promoted or demoted, or moved to another area or location.	2	
You have difficulties with your boss or another manager.	2	
You have difficulties with a colleague.	3	
You have a new boss.	2	
You are the only one of your race, sex or age-group at work.	2	
Your work is only commented on if it is unsatisfactory.	1	
You do not have enough work to do.	1	
You are not clear about what is expected of you.	2	
	Total score	

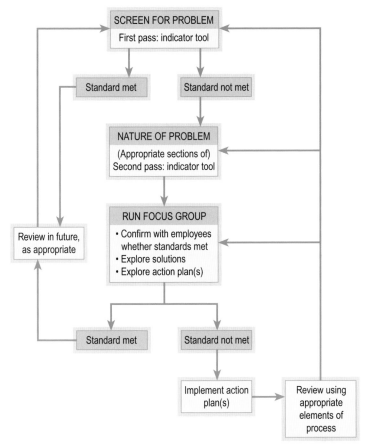

Figure 6.2   An adaptation of the HSE process of conducting a risk assessment for stress

Under 10: you are not over-stressed at work. You will be able to cope well with just about any eventuality that arises.

For Head Receptionists and Practice Managers, Figure 6.2 shows an adaptation of the HSE recommended approach to the process of conducting a risk assessment for stress in the practice.

STAGE 1	STAGE 2
Preparation	Second pass
■ Gaining management commitment	■ Defining problem areas in more detail
■ Raising employee awareness	Staff consultation
■ Selecting the pilot group	■ Consulting with employees (e.g. focus groups) to confirm the nature of the problem(s) and agree action required

(Continued)

STAGE 1	STAGE 2
First pass	Taking action
▪ Defining the current state of the organization against the management standards (i.e. given percentages)	▪ Interventions
▪ Feeding back results to staff and others	Review
	▪ Reviewing results
	▪ Dealing with individual issues

For further help and assistance with developing strategies to reduce stress in the workplace, contact the author (mac@daw.co.uk) or visit http://www.daw.co.uk

THE SYMPTOMS OF STRESS

Now look at the lists in Figure 6.3 and see how many of them apply to you. These are symptoms of stress and are the way your body tells you that you are too stressed.

Two or more symptoms from each of the lists means that you need to look at your life and find ways of minimizing the pressure by looking after yourself.

Figure 6.3 The physical and mental signs of stress

Physical signs		Mental signs	
Communicating less with other people (partner, friends or family)		Feeling of boredom and apathy	
Feeling tired and lacking in energy		Fears and phobias – heights, lifts, cars	
Being late for work or for other appointments more often		Preoccupation with your own health	
Putting on or losing more than 4.5kg (10 lb) in weight without meaning to		Fear of death, your own or other people's	
Eating for comfort, or not eating at all		Constant feeling of unease and anxiety	
Having trouble going to sleep, or staying asleep. Wanting to sleep all the time		Irritation with everybody	

(Continued)

Figure 6.3, Cont'd.   The physical and mental signs of stress

Physical signs		Mental signs	
Shortness of breath		Feeling unable to talk to anyone	
Indigestion, nausea or sickness		Inability to concentrate	
Frequent headaches		Reluctance to take a break or holiday	
Frequent minor ailments – colds, sore throats		Feeling that you aren't getting enough done	

Again, these are only meant to be guidelines and not a cue for panic – which would cause more stress!

If something stressful has just happened to you (perhaps you have just moved house, for instance) then you are bound to feel stressed and tired. This will decrease with time and, as long as you do not jump into another high stress situation immediately afterwards, you will probably be fine. You can't sit about doing nothing just in case it causes you stress!

STRESS REACTION TYPES

There are three basic stress types that one can identify depending on the way that individuals deal with stress.

Stress transmitters

People who are obviously under stress and unable to cope. Their inappropriate behaviours are infectious; they can cause a stress reaction in others who then become tense, anxious or irritable.

These 'transmitters' need to be guided on developing coping strategies. They also need to be made aware, in calm moments, that their behaviour has an impact on others that tends to fuel the stress build-up in the veterinary practice.

Stress dumpers

People who become stressed and get rid of it by 'dumping' their stress on to someone else. These people tend to walk away from the problem and pass it on to another to deal with.

They need to be made aware that they are employed to deal with problems. They may need help and guidance to develop the skills to deal with the problem rather than walk away. If it is a client problem that they walk away from, the guide in Chapters 7 and 8 may give them the pointers they need to deal with problems and complaints.

Stress carriers

People who just take the stress on board and get on as best they can. Stress carriers remember three key words – courage, tolerance and wisdom:

Courage to change that which can be changed…

Tolerance to accept that which cannot be changed…

And Wisdom to know the difference!

MINIMIZE YOUR OVERALL STRESS LEVELS

There are a number of things that you might like to consider to reduce your stress levels; ten are given below. Add these to your own list of ways to cope.

SHORT-TERM MEASURES

1. Make a list of the things you have to do and tick them off as you do them. It makes you feel more in control. Write them down 'with the end in mind'; by this is meant, rather than write: '*Phone Wholesaler*' write the purpose of the call, say: '*Get w'saler to agree credit note*'. A few more words but it clarifies the end point and makes the task clear – and perhaps less daunting!

2. Do the worst tasks first to get them over with – they are often never as bad as you thought anyway!

3. Rehearse things that you are dreading; ask yourself what would be the worst thing that could happen? Not much at work is exactly life-threatening!

4. Give yourself breaks – short 'breathers' – during the day whenever you can. Even a change of tasks can help. Remember how you feel when you stand back and admire a cleaned bathroom sink at home – all those shiny taps. Try a similar approach at work. Tidy a couple of feet of bookshelves. (Doing the whole lot at one go would not be possible and may in itself be stressful.) Tidy the reception area. Anything that is useful that creates a little order in your workspace can clear out stress.

5. Be clear about what is really important to you – animal welfare? So, even if the client is a 'pain', their pet deserves the best from the practice.

6. Keep a pet. Research shows that stroking an animal can reduce stress and the risk of heart disease. You probably do this already, yet working in veterinary practice and having to cope with the loss of pets and the clients' reaction all adds to stress.

7. Take it out on something inanimate. It may be a squash ball at the local squash club or, as one practice in West Yorkshire does, 'mug-a-mug'. They collect all the chipped mugs together in a cardboard box and when someone gets stressed, they take out a mug, go round to the big metal bins at the back of the practice and smash the mug into the bottom. No mess, no angry exchange of words, and stress is relieved.

8. Learn to say 'no'. This may be very difficult to say to clients – especially the more demanding. It may be even more difficult to say 'No' to your boss! So,

perhaps a more pragmatic approach might be to say, 'No, not yet'. We'll look at this again under 'assertiveness' later in this chapter.

9. Take a deep breath and count to ten before you deal with difficult situations. This allows the brain chemicals that gush out when we are alarmed to ebb away so that we can react in a more controlled fashion.

10. Don't bottle things up – get rid of your anger or frustration by talking to someone about it afterwards, and letting off steam. Remember, women tend to 'solve' a problem by talking about it, blokes just 'think it through'; we just need a little time!

There is also the three-phase model to consider in all situations where the demands of the job exceed the ability of the individual to cope:

Phase one: change your physical state

When the event is over and a convenient break occurs in the work, get away from the area and move to somewhere else, the rest room, an office, or the car park. Go and make a cup of tea. Not that you need the tea, perhaps, but the break from the physical state will do you good.

Phase two: change your emotional state

When you are taking the break, try to cool down. Calm yourself; this is where the 'count to ten' is so helpful in the immediate situation. For more substantial changes to the emotional state, you will need to take a longer break then ten seconds. While taking that break, think through the third phase.

Phase three: start to behave differently

Reconsider the high-pressure situation that led to the stress reaction you felt. What do you think you might do differently to avoid the situation occurring again? What help and support do you need in the practice to help you cope better next time? What must the organization of the practice address in order to prevent you having to cope with undue pressure over and above the usual demands of the job?

LONG-TERM RESILIENCE

While there are some things that you need to bring to the attention of your boss, there are also some things that we all can adopt to help ourselves. They are in three categories.

Physical resources

Whether these are adopting better relaxation and breathing techniques through such courses as Yoga or Pilates at the local sports centre or just raising your own awareness of the need to think about yourself, the benefits are an investment in yourself.

Healthy eating is not just a fad because, if you feel good, you can cope better and will suffer less of those irritating colds and so forth that just get you down.

Exercise goes hand in hand with healthy eating. Regular exercise does not have to be a penance – just try parking five minutes from the practice during the light summer months and enjoy the walk. Always remember the sound advice that you need to check with your GP if you take up strenuous exercise and you are not used to it.

Behavioural resources

Time management and being organized are fundamental. Make sure that you are familiar with all the systems and procedures in the practice and any efforts to reduce the number of mistakes and re-working or apologizing will save you hours in time.

Assertiveness training is also useful and is covered later in this chapter.

Communication skills are fundamental to reducing many of the stresses in veterinary practice both internally and with clients. Most of this book is about improved communication techniques.

Social resources

Balancing home and work is essential to get everything in proportion. You may have a work hard-play hard philosophy; provided you get the balance right there should be no problem. Those that work all hours and take their work home (even if only in their heads) are doing themselves and the practice no favours. Equally, being a party animal is fine if you have a private income; if you don't, remember to respect your employer and give the best of yourself through your shift and not take your tiredness out on your colleagues or clients.

A social-support network, both in the practice and at home, will be helpful to all concerned. Ask yourself, are you a solution seeker where you are always looking for someone else to solve your problems? Or are you a problem solver where you are always looking on the bright side of a situation and seeking to carry out what can be done rather than focusing on what cannot? If you are the latter, your social-support network will grow and you will have your positive attitude repaid with support.

ADVANCED STRESS MANAGEMENT

We have concentrated on helping to identify stress and to work on reducing its effects. However, it is also helpful to have some framework for identifying stress in other people and knowledge as to how to go about reducing the stress for them. This section deals with stress and the five 'drivers'.

The framework chosen is taken from Transactional Analysis[1], and has developed from the idea that each person creates his or her own life story. It is believed

[1] The basic idea of TA is that we relate to each other as 'child', 'adult', or 'parent' and it describes various 'ego' states. For more information on this subject, see Mackay, 2007b (Chapter 15–Self-Esteem).

that the story begins at birth, and is created out of all the experiences that affect the growing child. As a result of these experiences, the child develops a 'script' which becomes a life-plan. Clinical psychologists followed this idea that the script can be played out repetitively over very short time periods, and noticed that there were certain distinctive sets of behaviours which people seemed to move into just before they progressed to 'script' behaviour. These have been studied in depth and five of these behaviour sequences – called 'drivers' – are listed.

The significance of these for reducing stress is that, because when under stress it is difficult for us to remain entirely autonomous, those are the times when we fall into the behaviour determined by our life script. In other words, that is repetitive patterns of thinking, feeling and acting which were developed by us as a response to our early life experiences.

An important aspect of the way one's life script develops is that parents (and any other important figures of authority in relationship to the child) transmit values and standards to a growing child in a variety of ways. They may give direct instructions ('You must be kind and considerate to others'); they may model the behaviour (mother looks after the needs of family members); they may deprive or reward the child for certain behaviour (the child receives more smiles and hugs for certain types of behaviour). However they are transmitted, children are not able to understand the subtleties of these messages. They do not have the cognitive (thinking) ability to reflect upon and examine in depth the messages they are receiving. The young child is likely to receive any 'message' as a 'rule'. The child believes that she must do (or not do) whatever is being transmitted at the time. In time, these rules can become crystallized into rigid patterns of thinking, feeling and acting, which will emerge under stress. When we are not stressed we can decide whether the messages we carry in our head are appropriate for the present moment. But when we are under stress we feel as if we are driven by these rules. It seems as if we will only survive if we can be perfect/please/be strong/try hard/hurry up.

Figure 6.4 is a simple questionnaire designed to uncover your basic drivers. You may find that this is something that everyone in the practice might like to complete as it is as helpful to know what someone else's drivers are. If you know what other colleague's drivers are, you can develop approaches to help them cope with the pressure in reception and throughout the practice.

You will see that the questionnaire is divided into five sections. You will need to sum your score of the five questions in a section to give you your result. If you score 3½ or more in any section, this means that you have a *tendency* to exhibit this driver when placed under pressure. Figure 6.5 shows which questions relate to each of the five drivers.

It is quite possible that you may not score above 3½ in any section. Perhaps you have a tendency to not show your feelings in certain stressful situations and take things calmly. It may be that by talking about your assessment of yourself with another person who knows you well you may find that your

Figure 6.4   The 'Driver' Questionnaire revealing the extent to which you have a tendency to show any of the five drivers. Score yourself nil for a 'no', ½ for a 'to some extent' and 1 for a 'yes'.

Driver questionnaire			
This questionnaire is not a 'personality test'. It is intended to stimulate your self-awareness and indicate the kind of stress behaviour you may typically or frequently get into. Answer questions 'yes', 'no', or 'to some extent' – if you feel that the statement is a little like you, on occasions, maybe at home or at work, then answer 'to some extent'. Definitely you or not you: answer accordingly...			
	No	To some extent	Yes
1. Do you set yourself high standards (of achievement or success) then mentally criticize yourself for failing to meet them?			
2. Is it important for you to be right?			
3. Do you feel discomforted (e.g. annoyed, irritated) by small messes or discrepancies such as a spot on a garment, picture crooked, an ornament or tool out of place, a disorderly presentation of work?			
4. Do you hate to be interrupted?			
5. Do you like to explain things in detail and precisely?			
6. Do you do things, especially for others, that you don't really want to do but you find yourself doing them anyway?			
7. Is it important to you to be liked?			
8. Are you fairly easily persuaded?			
9. Do you dislike being 'different'?			
10. Do you dislike conflict?			
11. Do you have a tendency to do a lot of things simultaneously?			
12. Would you describe yourself as 'quick' and find yourself getting impatient with others?			
13. Do you tend to talk at the same time as others, or finish their sentences for them?			
14. Do you like to 'get on with the job' rather than talk about it?			
15. Do you set unrealistic time limits (especially too short)?			
16. Do you hide or control your feelings?			

(Continued)

Figure 6.4, Cont'd. The 'Driver' Questionnaire revealing the extent to which you have a tendency to show any of the five drivers. Score yourself nil for a 'no', ½ for a 'to some extent' and 1 for a 'yes'. Total your scores in five sections, see Fig. 6.5.

17. Are you reluctant to ask for help?			
18. Do you have a tendency to put yourself (or find yourself) in the position of being depended upon?			
19. Do you have a tendency not to realize how tired, or hungry, or ill you are, but instead 'keep going'?			
20. Do you prefer to do things on your own?			
21. Do you hate 'giving up' or 'giving in', always hoping that this time it will work?			
22. Do you have a tendency to start things and not finish them?			
23. Do you tend to compare yourself (or your performance) with others and feel better than or worse than them accordingly?			
24. Do you find yourself going round in circles with a problem, feeling stuck but unable to let go of it?			
25. Do you tend to be 'the rebel' or 'odd one out' in a group?			

opinion of yourself may be reviewed in the light of their experience of you. Don't worry about having a low score in all sections, it just means that you cope as well as anyone else with pressure and do not exhibit a strong driver in any particular direction; you will be less predictable in how you are likely to respond to stress.

Figure 6.5 The five 'drivers' and how they relate to the questionnaire in Figure 6.4

Questions	Driver
1–5	Be perfect
6–10	Please
11–15	Hurry up
16–20	Be strong
21–25	Try hard

If you have scored over 3½ in any section then you have a tendency to exhibit that driver. Refer to the appropriate section below for further information about the driver, how to help yourself cope with stress, and how to help others cope if they too have the driver.

You may have more than one driver – even all five. Having more than one means that you may be quite flexible in the way that you respond to stressful situations, although with three or more drivers some may say unpredictable! It means that you have developed a variety of scripts to deal with stress and may have to look to a variety of coping strategies to reduce the impact of stress on you.

BE PERFECT

Language and appearance clues: these words and phrases are often used by people when they are in the grip of a Be Perfect driver: 'as it were', 'probably', 'possibly', 'certainly', 'completely', 'one might say'. They speak in completed sentences, perhaps numbering off various points. Their dress is usually very coordinated and elegant. Their language and their appearance are all indications of their desire to be perfect.

Characteristics: each driver carries positive characteristics, as well as negative ones, and persons influenced by this driver will be purposeful, moral and have very high standards. They will be task-oriented and extremely logical, and very good at seeing the best way of achieving the success or completion of a task.

Stress caused by: anything which indicates the danger of loss of control; for instance other people's perceived 'low' standards or illogicality; over-emotionalism from other people; failure to achieve goals.

Stress behaviour: as the pressure and therefore stress increases, the person will become more and more single-minded, seeing only their own point of view. They will become more and more controlling. They may become very arrogant and aggressive in arguments and will not be able to take account of other people's different views. They will be focused on the goal and so may discount the people around. They will communicate predominantly in 'thought' language and be very uncomfortable at displays of extreme emotion.

Ways of reducing the pattern of stress in self

Be willing to appreciate different values held by other people rather than just seeing your own as valuable.

1. List down all your personal values and give them a rating, with a high mark for the most important and lower marks as their importance decreases. Then work out how to respond appropriately. When under stress the tendency is to treat everything as important and so energy is poured into issues that are actually in themselves not important.

2. Become more conscious of your tendency to be self-righteous and to respond to people in a parental manner, and make a point of communicating your feelings.
3. Be willing to laugh at yourself.

Helping to reduce stress in others

These are the kind of interventions which will help to reduce the stress in someone who is responding to their Be Perfect driver.

1. Reassurance that they 'are not to blame' for everyone else's failings.
2. Be punctual and keep agreements with them.
3. Never discount their worries or attention to detail.
4. If you have a difference of opinion express your own values with conviction – and logically.
5. If you have to confront them, do it gently, firmly and calmly.
6. Show appreciation of their achievements, e.g. 'That report you produced is excellent'.
7. Give them the facts, rather than forcing them to talk about their emotions.

PLEASE

Language and appearance clues: a characteristic language pattern is to start off a sentence positively and end it negatively, e.g. 'It really is a wonderful day, but these kind of days often end in rain.' 'This is a really good course, but I don't know how I'm going to remember everything.' Statements are turned into questions by phrases like, 'Is that OK with you?'; '...kind of...?'; 'What do you think about...?' The tone of voice is often high, rising at the end of each sentence. The person with a strong Please driver will make a lot of effort to look attractive and dress 'prettily' rather than neatly, wearing jewellery and perfume to complete the effect.

Characteristics: the person with a strong Please driver loves spending time with other people, and is comfortable in social situations. They are usually skilled in dealing with others, and like to look after people. They are as pleasant as possible to everyone; are extremely law-abiding and helpful; concerned with doing the right thing.

Distress caused by: being ignored; being criticized; their fear is that they will be rejected by being found 'blameworthy'.

Stress behaviour: these persons will become more and more emotional, and will not respond to demands to 'be logical'. Their language becomes peppered with clichés and, if the stress increases, they will be unable to say 'no' to anyone. One of the most destructive aspects of this stress pattern is the urge to rescue anyone and everyone. Obviously, if there is an emergency then taking charge is often the wisest thing to do. If there is no emergency, then rescuing (which is defined as doing something that has not been asked for, or doing more than your share) will, in the long term, not really help the other person. Every time you do something for someone, that person is deprived of the opportunity to do it him or herself and learn from that action.

Ways of reducing stress pattern in self

1. The person with a strong Please driver does feel responsible for other people, and expects them to reciprocate by taking responsibility for their wellbeing. So, in order to break through this, it is important to be willing to accept responsibility for what happens to you and what you do to others.
2. Listen carefully to others, and respond to what they are actually saying, rather than to what you believe they want.
3. Develop autonomy – become content with what you do for yourself, rather than just for other people.

Helping to reduce stress in others

1. Thank them politely for their help – but try not to be too gushing as that will only reinforce the driver.
2. Stay near the surface of communication, unless you are able and willing to cope with the amount of emotion that may be uncovered.
3. Never lose your temper – you may say something particularly hurtful that later you'd regret.
4. If you are angry, express your feelings politely.
5. If you have to confront them, do it with patience.
6. Give no strokes for clichés (where they don't actually say anything, they are just trying to be nice); stroke abundantly for authentic communication (when they give genuine opinions, for example).
7. Acknowledge them for being the person they are. 'I really enjoy working with you'; 'It's lovely having you in the team'. This is different from the acknowledgement for the Be Perfect, which is primarily for what they have achieved. If you say, 'That report you did was really good', the Please person will be thinking, 'But does she really like me?'

Hurry up

Language and appearance clues: words and phrases like 'quick', 'get going', 'hurry up', 'don't waste time', 'there's no time to…'. The overriding impression of someone in the grip of a Hurry Up driver is that they are in a hurry! They may speak very rapidly and will usually be doing more than one thing at a time. Gestures like finger-tapping, foot tapping, wriggling about in the chair, constant checking of watch are also indications.

Characteristics: this person will be lively; adventurous; excited; often described as the 'life and soul of the party'; enthusiastic; quick with a capacity for doing lots of things at once.

Distress caused by: time to think; silence; having 'nothing to do'.

Stress behaviour: as the stress increases activity will become more and more frenetic.

Reduction of stress in self

1. Learn to love life for its own sake, so that the fear that life has no meaning is less threatening.
2. A greater feeling of security will arise if you develop a belief system – what is more important: the speed of life or the quality of life?
3. Realize that you do not need to earn love by proving how much you can do.
4. Practise your empathy and listening skills.
5. Be on time by not fitting in 'just one more thing' before your appointment.
6. Make the time to express appreciation of other people.
7. Make lists; create structures and order despite how you feel about them.

Helping to reduce pattern of stress in others

1. Praise for efficiency – not speed.
2. Enjoy their spontaneity.
3. Never be intimidated by their outbursts.
4. Don't say thanks for the speed at which they work; or for the ability to do several things at once.
5. Stroke for taking time. 'I really appreciate how much time you are giving to this'; 'Take as much time as you need'; 'It's good to see you slowing down'.

BE STRONG

Language and appearance clues: the Be Strong is concerned with not appearing vulnerable, so language tends to be distanced from feelings. 'That makes me sad', rather than 'I feel sad'. Words like 'one', 'us', 'we', 'it', are used to replace 'I'. Face and body tend to be immobile – another indication of the urge to hide any evidence of feelings which may mean weakness.

Characteristics: the Be Strong driver carries characteristics like self-sufficiency, helpfulness, reliability. People who have a dominant 'Be Strong' driver enjoy tasks which are repetitive and like working on their own. They are extremely stoical in the face of difficulties and will carry on regardless.

Stress caused by: the fear of rejection through being seen as vulnerable, being 'forced' to say what they feel; exposing their weaknesses.

Stress behaviour: when under stress the Be Strong driver leads to rather withdrawn, withholding behaviour. The person becomes quieter and quieter and reluctant to communicate. It is as if every word has to be dragged out. The conversation tends to sound this way. 'Is there anything wrong?' 'No', 'Are you sure?' No answer. 'I can see something is wrong – what is it?' No answer. The questioner becomes more like an interrogator, trying to get a response.

Ways of reducing the stress pattern in self

Learn to take as well as give. The Be Strong are generous givers – always ready to help. It is as if by being this way they will never have to reveal their own needs. Even up the balance, so that you are not covering your own needs, and be willing to express them.

Helping to reduce stress in others

1. Praise them for consideration and kindness, because they often get taken for granted.
2. Give them a surprise treat.
3. Do not be effusive.
4. Use irony; 'I must say – you are the most unreliable person'.
5. Don't force them into expressions of vulnerability.
6. Don't shout, or they will retreat even further.
7. If you want something done, give them clear instructions. Tell them exactly what you want done, e.g. 'I would like this report typed on A4 sheets, with all the corrections as marked. Please let me have it on Friday morning, and if there are any problems telephone me to discuss them'.

Try hard

Language and appearance clues: often the person in a Try Hard driver will use the word 'try'. 'Yes, I'll try to get it finished'; 'I am trying my best...'. When it is used in this way it usually means 'I'll try to do it instead of actually doing it'. Other typical words and phrases are: 'can't', 'I don't understand', 'it's very difficult...'. Often the person appears very tense, maybe frowning or with fists clenched.

Characteristics: intense and committed to righting wrongs; usually on the side of the underdog and is often a worker for political or other causes; passionate; takes on lots of tasks – often doesn't complete them; sets high goals – often not achieved; very hard worker.

Distress caused by: being criticized for not caring or for being irresponsible; being told 'You're not trying'; for perceived irresponsibility in others.

Stress behaviour: one of the main effects is that much effort goes into trying, but very little is achieved. Lots of tasks may be taken on, and promises be made, but something always seems to get in the way of a success. One of the problems for someone with a Try Hard driver is that if their belief is that they are only acceptable if they try hard, how will they be able to survive when they have succeeded! It is as if it becomes more important to go on trying than to finish. The person tends to move into reactive, rebellious behaviour.

Ways of reducing pattern of stress in self

1. Notice how often you use the word 'Try', say instead 'I will' or 'I won't'.
2. Before you take on extra work, check that it is realistic for you to do so. If your schedule is full, decide what you will give up in order to take on the new job. Check also that you want to do it as opposed to believing that you ought to.

3. Be willing to distinguish between things you can and cannot change.
4. Stop comparing yourself to others.
5. Create standards for yourself, which are not related to others.
6. Start now not tomorrow.

Helping to reduce stress in others

1. If the person is being very competitive, ignore it. Don't get involved in arguments that are focused on comparisons, e.g. 'You don't understand as much as I do'; 'They are not working hard enough'.
2. Never let them off what they committed themselves to do. If you do, the implication is that you don't expect them to succeed.
3. Do not stroke for trying, stroke for finishing.

SUMMARY

In this section, you have looked briefly at your overall stress levels at work, whether you are suffering from the symptoms of over-stress and at ways of keeping your stress levels down in the short term and ways of building long-term resiliance. You have also explored the five basic 'drivers' – now you may understand yourself better, what of your work colleagues, what are their drivers? If you get them to do the questionnaire, too, you may be able to help others limit the down-side of their drivers!

The next section focuses on how you can control your negative reactions in difficult situations.

SELF-TALK OR NLP (NEURO-LINGUISTIC PROGRAMMING)

Shut your eyes for a few seconds and try not to think of anything in particular.

You will find that your head is full of pictures, words, sentences, sensations and sounds. This 'babble' goes on all the time. Your brain talks to you constantly about the world around you. It filters it and makes sense of it in your own terms. Most of the time you are not aware of the process, but without it you would be confronted with an orchestra of sights, sounds and sensations with no pattern or meaning.

Imagine a toddler going into a room full of noisy people for the very first time. He or she does not know what to make of it. That is how confused you would be without your self-talk to interpret the world for you.

NLP Theory: NLP is a profoundly different effective 'how-to' technology for personal excellence. NLP is based on the study of the most influential components involved in shaping our experiences.

Neuro-Linguistic Programming (NLP) has many strengths, but a clear and helpful name isn't one of them! Fortunately, it can be defined straightforwardly as the *study of excellence.*

Neuro – the unique way we translate the information we receive through our senses about the external world and what is happening around us, and how this translation affects the way we think, our physiology, how we feel and how we behave.

Linguistic – How we express our experience to ourselves and to others through the language we use and how the language we use affects our experience, behaviour and feelings.

Programming – How habitual, often unconscious, patterns of thoughts and feelings develop through the course of our lives affect our current behaviour – and how these patterns can be changed.

People do not react directly to situations; Figure 6.6 shows what really happens. Your 'self-talk' tells you about the situation, and how to feel about it. As a result of how you feel, you act.

Sometimes, when your self-talk is positive, it will work for you, but sometimes, when the self-talk is negative, it will work against you. For example, if you tell yourself that your client will be unfriendly or difficult, what is likely to happen? (Figure 6.7.)

Once you are aware of your negative messages, you can control them. One technique is to say 'stop'! out loud to yourself when you catch yourself being negative; then immediately find a positive statement, and say it to yourself. It helps to have some positive statements ready. It may sound odd, but it does work.

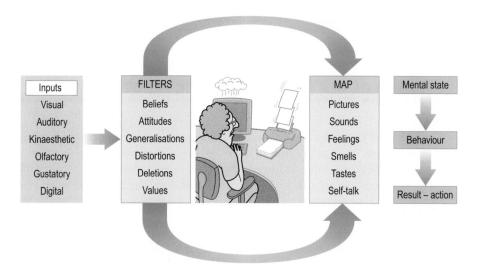

Figure 6.6   A diagram showing how our various sensory inputs are filtered by experience to leave us with a chosen 'map' defining our mental state that in turn affects our chosen behaviour and actions.

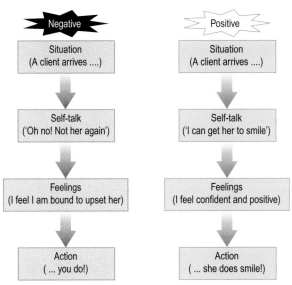

Figure 6.7   How negative or positive self-talk tends towards outcomes that are either negative or positive: we have a choice...!

Self-talk, either positive or negative, goes on before, during and after an event – you can choose which to use. It is up to you to turn your negative messages into positive ones.

Remember, identifying the things that bring us success is a better approach to achievement in life and work than focusing on problems. Unfortunately, childhood teaches us not to boast and that pride comes before a fall, and that happiness is no more than a short step to smugness; all these qualities can be related to complacency and our achievements slip into the background of continued struggle. The warning is that 'the caution that informs our perceptions can be self-fulfilling...be careful what you look for – you might just find it...if you look for problems, you will find them'. Conversely: 'a focus on success is more likely to generate positive results...'. For more ideas on 'Achievement' and the power of positive thinking, see Mackay (2007b).

SECTION SUMMARY

You can choose how you view a particular situation and you can either say something positive to yourself or something negative – this is called neuro-linguistic programming and your behaviour and actions relate directly to this. Turn your negative messages into positive ones.

TAKING THE STRESS OUT OF DIFFICULT SITUATIONS

The essential ingredient of excellent client service, and of good relationships, is to make your client feel special by treating them with:

T	R	U	S	T
R	E	N	E	R
U	S	D	N	U
T	P	E	S	S
H	E	R	I	T
F	C	S	T	
U	T	T	I	
L		A	V	
N		N	I	
E		D	T	
S		I	Y	
S		N		
		G		

Review Chapter 4 if you have not read it recently as a reminder. We will look at client service solutions in Chapter 8 but, for now, we'll focus on a few ideas to help with the pressure at work

TAKE IT PROFESSIONALLY

When you are dealing with a difficult client or an awkward situation, this still applies. However, there is one more vital element to be added:

When you are under attack – *Take it professionally not personally.*

This is easier to say than to do, but it is not impossible, and it is a skill well worth making an effort to develop. Taking things professionally, not personally, means developing a professional personality to protect you from the kind of upset which might make you feel miserable and defeated by the job. Being aware of the difference between being professional and taking it personally will help you to sharpen your skills and to speed the process of learning.

1. Remember that it is part of your job!
   One way of reminding yourself, if you are faced with a sticky situation with a client (or with a difficult colleague or superior, for that matter) is to take a deep breath and say something like this to yourself:
   'I am being paid to do this job. That means that I am a professional. I make my living by dealing with clients to a veterinary practice. Sometimes it is not easy, sometimes it is frustrating and sometimes I have to deal with difficult behaviours from people. I can make it easier for myself by keeping a sense of perspective and by being professional.'
2. Focus on the problem, not the people. There is a school of thought that there is no such thing as difficult people – but their behaviour might be!
3. Another way you can help you do this is to keep the focus away from yourself and on the problem at hand.

This means that you need to keep your mind on the solution, not on the personalities involved. Ask yourself what the problem is, and how it can be solved. Figure 6.8 may give you some ideas.

4. Involve another person.

When you find yourself in a difficult situation you don't know how to handle, or you are facing an angry client and you are at your wits' end, involve someone else. Never let an incident get out of hand because you do not know what to do, or because you have let yourself become too involved or upset. Even if you are the only one on duty at that time – get someone else (one of the vets) on the phone if need be.

It is often (but not always) the case that a different face can defuse a client's anger. They have taken their frustration out on you, and someone else can take over and sort it out. It is not fair, but it is part of being on the 'front line' – sometimes you have to take the flack.

If you feel yourself getting angry or upset, involving someone else is the best and most professional way of resolving it, because no one ever wins an argument with a client, so it is not worth letting one develop.

HANDLING SITUATIONS OBJECTIVELY

Can you think of a time, in work or outside work, when something happened, you took it personally, and became upset?

The example below will give you a start:

- What was the situation?
  A man who became abusive when I asked him to wait in the queue.
- How did you react?
  I tried to explain, but got upset when he shouted at me. Other clients were waiting to be seen for their appointment, I felt I couldn't cope.
- What happened to end it?
  A colleague went to find the practice manager who came to calm him down.
- How did you feel afterwards?
  Upset. I felt a fool in front of the manager.
- Is there any way you could have handled it better? How could you have reacted?

Figure 6.8   Use positive self-talk to focus not on the problem but on the solution

Rather than thinking:	⇨	Think instead:
This person is accusing me of this mistake	⇨	How can we solve this problem?
She is a really grumpy old witch	⇨	How can I deal with her efficiently and move on?
I wasn't on duty that day	⇨	What can we (the practice) learn from this?
She or he can't treat me like that	⇨	What needs to be done?
It's not my fault	⇨	It's my job to find a way to make things better.

After I'd explained, I could have asked him to wait while I got help, or I could have asked a vet to explain to him first to avoid trouble.

- How might you have felt afterwards?
  I might have felt that I'd been able to handle the situation, felt capable and not been so upset afterwards.
- What have I learnt from this?
  In that case, you must find someone to talk to about it, do not blame yourself, and remember:

There are some people you just cannot please.

We have looked at dealing with difficult situations and difficult people so far.

However, sometimes situations develop which do not just involve a single client, or particularly difficult ones. People have different ways of coping with busy times.

In most jobs facing the public, it is essential to keep up the standard of respect and understanding of clients while also being fast and efficient. There is one situation where this is especially true, that of the busy reception with the phone going all the time, a queue of people coming and going, and vets asking for the world! Let us turn to queue management.

QUEUE MANAGEMENT

The chances are that if you feel under stress and show it, your clients will react badly. If you can stay calm and pleasant, you will reassure them and keep the process running smoothly. Even the best laid plans of your appointment system will fail through the (reasonable) unexpected. This includes people being off sick, or called away to an emergency. Giving the people the right information and offering some alternatives will be crucial.

Go through the checklist in Figure 6.9, answering honestly, how do you react?

All these suggestions are easy to put into practice when business is quiet. But when it is busy and you are under pressure, the strain can begin to show. Remember that:

Figure 6.9   Checklist: for queue management

Do you:	
Smile at each client?	❑
Make eye contact?	❑
Show them that you have noticed they are waiting?	❑
Apologize to each client for keeping them waiting when it is their turn?	❑
Acknowledge each client with a smile or nod of your head if you are busy?	❑
Explain what the delay is in a friendly manner?	❑

- it takes no more time to smile than it does to frown
- a gesture of acknowledgement makes clients feel they matter
- showing your irritation only makes you more irritated
- being rude or off-hand makes clients more impatient and angry
- efficiency is the same as giving good service
- most people just want some information on why there is a delay
- most people will feel better if you acknowledge how frustrating the delay must be for them
- you would prefer to be treated with courtesy in their place.

At the end of the day, it is likely that queue management problems may not be something that you can address directly yourself. It may be that the practice managers or partners need to be made aware of the suboptimal resources and do something about it to stop business being lost.

SECTION SUMMARY

There are three ways that you can deal with difficult situations:

- Remembering that it is part of your job, and being professional.
- Concentrating on the problem, not the personalities.
- Involving someone else.

We also looked at ways to improve on your client care skills when you are busy.

BEHAVING ASSERTIVELY

In the last section, you saw that it helps to be objective in difficult situations. The most effective way of coping with difficult or unpleasant clients is to be assertive. Being assertive means establishing your control within a situation but without being overbearing or avoiding the situation altogether. It is a difficult balance to achieve but, once you do it, you will feel much more confident. You will have discovered an inner resource that can help you overcome stress and stay professional no matter what pressures you face.

In this section, we will look at how to evaluate our own level of assertiveness while, in Chapter 7, we will explore assertive behaviour in more detail as it affects our ability to 'profit from complaints'.

AGGRESSIVE, ASSERTIVE AND PASSIVE BEHAVIOUR

Assertive behaviour is usually defined in relation to aggressive and passive behaviour.

Aggressive behaviour is when someone behaves in an overbearing, unpleasant and sometimes menacing way. They are so determined to get their own way that they bully others into saying 'yes', often unconsciously. People often behave aggressively when they feel that they are under pressure; when the stress gets on top of them. Aggressive behaviour in this situation is usually not a choice but a natural response to a pressurized situation. A client might not blame you for behaving aggressively when you are obviously under pressure, but they won't like it either.

Passive behaviour, in contrast, is often the style of a shy or unconfident person. A passive person will tend to hold back their opinions and keep quiet. They may end up following the group or saying 'yes' to someone else's idea because they do not have the strength of character to make their own views known. Someone who is anxious or does not want to draw attention to themselves may behave passively in order to try to minimize the stress they feel. However, passive behaviour can allow stress to build up inside. If you don't express your real feelings, they may burst out at some unexpected moment.

Neither aggressive nor passive behaviour is an effective way to behave with clients, or in fact, anyone. Aggressive behaviour will irritate clients. A client who is bullied or snapped at will not be eager to return. Passive behaviour may also turn people off. A client who gets little guidance or response will be disappointed and not impressed with the service they receive.

Aggressive and passive responses are not effective coping strategies. They will increase the stress you feel rather than relieving it.

The key is to be assertive: to keep control in a stressful situation by expressing your views and intentions but also continue to listen to the client and respond.

So, how assertive are you?

Most of us need some help in being assertive, even if we already have some of the qualities and skills required. (Chapter 7 explores assertiveness in more detail)

The quiz in Figure 6.10 gives you a chance to test how assertive you are.

Look at the comments below to see how assertive you are.

Figure 6.10   Quiz: test how assertive you are

1. A friend insists that you have dinner with them, but you are very tired. Do you:	✓
a) let yourself be persuaded?	❑
b) say 'no' outright?	❑
c) go along but make it clear that you don't want to be there?	❑
d) explain that you are tired, say you can't make it that night but fix another date?	❑
2. Your boss suggests that you have not been working as hard as you should. You disagree. Do you:	
a) keep quiet and accept the judgement?	❑
b) engage in a fierce argument to state your position?	❑
c) explain your case calmly, giving evidence?	❑
d) resign then and there and threaten to take your supervisor to an industrial tribunal?	❑

Figure 6.10, Cont'd.   Quiz: test how assertive you are

3. In a restaurant the waiter keeps on telling you that he will be with you in a minute. Fifteen minutes go by and you will be late for your next appointment. Do you:	
a) get up and walk out of the restaurant?	❑
b) continue to wait while your blood pressure rises?	❑
c) call the person you will be meeting to explain the situation?	❑
d) ask to speak to the manager?	❑
4. Your train is delayed and no information is given to explain why. Do you:	
a) sit calmly and wait since the situation is out of your control?	❑
b) make an effort to find an attendant for further information?	❑
c) pull the emergency cord to get some attention?	❑
d) sit waiting in irritation, unable to concentrate on anything else?	❑
5. You have bought a ticket which gives you train and bus travel for the day. You use it on the train, but when you get on a bus, the conductor tells you that the ticket is invalid. Do you:	
a) storm off the bus and decide to walk instead?	❑
b) explain that you're sure the ticket is valid asking if he'll reconsider? If not, you get off and walk?	❑
c) agree to pay the excess fare-it's easier than arguing?	❑
d) ask who you can contact to report the situation?	❑
6. A client returns an item to you and complains that it is defective. He is very abusive about the quality of the product and you find him unpleasant. Do you:	
a) give him his money back and ignore his comments?	❑
b) express genuine concern, give him a replacement and refer the fault to the manufacturer?	❑
c) snap at him in irritation and refuse to refund his purchase?	❑
d) refer him to your manager?	❑

Situation 1

a) This is a passive response – you are taking the easy option, but you probably won't have a good time.
b) This response borders on assertive–aggressive. You succeed in making your views known, but will probably hurt your friend's feelings.
c) This is an aggressive response – no one will have a good time.
d) This is an assertive response. You achieve the best end for all parties concerned. No one ends up doing what they don't want to do.

Situation 2

a) A passive response – you are suppressing your feelings, perhaps out of fear?
b) Probably an aggressive response which will not win over your supervisor.
c) An assertive response. If your supervisor resists, you may have cause to refer the matter above him or her.
d) A bullying, aggressive response which will achieve nothing.

Situation 3

a) An assertive–aggressive response. You make your views known through your actions and are in control, but will continue to feel irritated after the event.
b) A passive response.
c) A pragmatic response which is ultimately passive at heart.
d) An assertive response. The action may prompt an instant response from the waiter. It will also make you feel and be more in control.

Situation 4

a) A passive response. If you are lucky enough to be able to remain calm, you may not suffer much stress, but you are not in control.
b) An assertive response. You are making a move towards gaining control.
c) An aggressive response which will not help.
d) A passive–aggressive response. You are doing nothing except getting yourself tied up in knots of frustration.

Situation 5

a) An aggressive response. You overreact without trying to reason or find out more.
b) An assertive response. You have done as much as you can in the situation. Your next step might be to write a letter of complaint.
c) A passive response. You accept the conductor's authority even though you know it is wrong.
d) An assertive response which may prompt him to accept your ticket but will at least give you access to a possible refund.

Situation 6

a) A passive response. Perhaps the path of least resistance given the situation.
b) An assertive response. He will leave, feeling that his views have been heard and responded to. You have behaved as professionally as possible under the circumstances.
c) An aggressive response which could cost you your job.
d) A passive–assertive response. It may be your only choice in the situation but looks like 'copping out'.

You should use the results of this exercise to decide whether you need to be more assertive. You can feed your findings into an action plan for yourself (see the Appendix).

In most of these situations, you were the client. In the last one, though, you were serving a difficult client. Assertive behaviour will give you the authority to deal with difficult clients. It will also keep your blood pressure down and help you stay free of stress and be professional under pressure.

SECTION SUMMARY
In this section, you have seen the differences between aggressive, assertive and passive behaviour. Assertive behaviour helps you stay professional no matter how much stress you are facing.

You have reviewed whether you are already assertive or not. This information will help you plan actions to take, to make sure you stay professional under pressure.

KEY TIPS FOR STAYING PROFESSIONAL UNDER PRESSURE

- Keep your stress levels down – look after yourself.
- Events don't make you upset –your self-talk does that.
- You can control your reactions.
- Tell yourself to stop! and be positive.
- Turn negative self-talk into positive 'self-talk'
  a) before the event
  b) during the event
  c) after the event.
- Take it professionally, not personally.
- Remember that it is part of your job!
- Focus on the problem, not the people.
- Involve another person, if necessary.
- No one ever wins an argument with a client.
- Apologize for any inconvenience.
- Remember – there are some people you just cannot please!
- It takes no more time to smile than to frown.
- Be assertive, not aggressive or passive.
- Use assertiveness to control difficult situations and stay professional.
- Assertiveness relieves stress.

References

Mackay, A.R. (2007a) Recruitment, Retention, & Releasing People. Butterworth Heinemann

Mackay, A.R. (2007b) Motivation, Ability & Confidence Building in People. Butterworth Heinemann

Health and Safety Statistics Highlights 2001/02. Available at: http://www.hse.gov.uk/statistics/overall/hssh0102.pdf . With supporting material available from links within this document and via the HSE statistics web page. Available at: http://www.hse.gov.uk/statistics/index.htm

HSE information sheet 2/99/EMSU. Economic impact: Revised data from the self-reported work-related illness survey in 1995 (SWI95). Available at http://www.hse.gov.uk/statistics/2002/ecimpact.pdf

Smith, A., Brice, C., Collins, A., Matthews, V. and McNamara, R. (2000) The Scale of Occupational Stress: a further analysis of the impact of demographic factors and type of job. CRR 311/2000. HSE Books. Available at: http://www.hse.gov.uk/research/crr_pdf/2000/crr00311.pdf

Chapter 7
Profit from complaints

Clients will let you know how you are doing dealing with them – or their pets – in three ways: compliments, comments and complaints. All three are worth noting – all perhaps written down – as they act as pointers to what's going right or wrong within your practice.

We all hear and remember compliments – although they sometimes seem to be far less common than the other two! But more negative comments – even the briefest remarks made in the waiting room – are worth your attention too. They can be useful early warning signs of dissatisfaction or a 'glitch' in the system, and a small concern neglected can soon fester into a full-blown complaint and take up more time and energy than if the practice had addressed it at the comment stage. Obviously, whoever receives a complaint is the client's first point of contact for the client. If it is you and you seem genuinely concerned and interested in helping to resolve the matter, you'll win respect both for yourself and for your practice.

Handling complaints on behalf of your practice takes sensitivity and tact from you – especially when you find yourself on the receiving end of an unwelcome verbal attack from some irate client. Naturally enough, it also takes skill and professionalism.

Not surprisingly, no one likes to deal with complaints, whether the criticism is about them or about the organization they work for. In an ideal world, there would be no complaints. It is not an ideal world, though, and people do complain, especially clients!

It therefore makes sense to use the opportunity constructively – to see a complaint as a second chance to get it right.

Research has shown that:

- Most dissatisfied customers do not complain. The average business does not hear from 96% of its unhappy customers.
- For every complaint received there will be another 26 customers with problems – at least six of these will be serious.
- Complaints are not made because people think it's not worth the time and effort, they don't know how or where to complain, or they believe the practice would be indifferent to them.
- Non-complainers are the least likely group to buy from the practice again. A complainer who gets a response is more likely to come back. Between 65 and 90% of non-complainers will never buy from you again and you will never know why.

It is better to have complaints than silent dissatisfaction! You need to keep in close touch with your customers' feelings to ensure that they remain customers! So, learning how to receive, respond and turn complaints round is vital.

FURTHER DEVELOPMENTS ON POSITIVE THINKING

In Chapter 6 we were introduced to NLP – Neuro-Linguistic Programming. This and subsequent sections explore the power of positive thinking further – particularly in respect of dealing with complaints.

Whether these complaints come by phone or in person, they are always upsetting for the staff who have to handle them. Because support staff are more likely to be on-hand at the time, they are the ones who usually take the brunt of the complaint. It is often true that a complaint made to support staff is more vicious than when it is made to veterinary staff. And it is often the case that a complaint is nastier when made by phone than when it is made in person.

How often have you warned a vet that a tiger is on the warpath, only to find that when it arrives, it's only a kitten? It may be something you, or somebody else in the practice, have said or done. It may be a complete misunderstanding, or it may be a genuinely justifiable complaint. But don't forget, the reason you are confronted with an angry client may have nothing to do with the practice, or anything that has happened within it. Sometimes you will have no way of knowing the circumstances that lie behind it. Try never to pre-judge the issue. All that should matter is that, in the end, you retain the client, and the client wants to return to the practice. Leave decisions about never wanting to see them again to your employer.

As a general rule, by way of introduction to the subject, whether on the phone or in person, serious complaints are better handled in private – whenever possible. Try to arrange that your side of such telephone conversations, or an interview with a client, does not take place in the hearing of a waiting room full of other clients, all eager to learn the juicy details. Transfer the call to a phone in an office, or show a client into a vacant consulting room or office. Do it politely, but don't explain why. They may prefer that the whole world hear what they have to say. They will certainly say they do. Try to remain calm, and always polite. Try to be helpful. Stick to facts yourself, and try to encourage the client to do the same. Take responsibility, but not the blame.

Further ideas can be found on a very useful document; type the following onto your web browser:

http://www.bsava.com/VirtualContent/85242/complaints_procedure_vds.pdf

So let us now turn to some positive thinking about complaints.

POSITIVE THINKING!

In this section, you will evaluate your current skill level for dealing with complaints and pinpoint areas for improvement.

How well do you deal with complaints? Figure 7.1 is a straightforward self-assessment quiz.

Figure 7.1   Quiz: Do you have positive thinking when you deal with complaints?

Are you:	✓
1. Always pleasant to customers even if they are not pleasant to you?	☐
2. Always ready to welcome suggestions from customers and from your manager about how you could improve in your job?	☐
3. Able to receive and handle complaints, without feeling personally attacked?	☐
4. Able to smile when you don't feel like it?	☐
5. Always able to apologize to a client, even if it is not your fault?	☐
6. Willing to listen carefully and sympathetically and find out what they want?	☐
7. Able to give reasons and positive suggestions when you can't do exactly what the client wants?	☐
8. Able to keep calm and behave professionally if a client becomes upset?	☐
9. Able to calm a client if necessary, and involve someone else if you become upset?	☐
10. Able to recover and profit from complaints and ensure that the client goes away feeling that you were helpful, you solved the problem satisfactorily, and wanting to return?	☐

Scoring

- It is very difficult to get ten ticks on the checklist in Figure 7.1. If you have, you must be a perfect professional, with few faults and a great deal of experience. However, there is still bound to be something for you in this chapter, despite your high score!
- 8–9 ticks: Almost perfect. You are confident and positive and able to cope well with difficult situations.
- 6–7 ticks: Good. This means that you are good at your job. A little more work on it would not go amiss.
- 4–5 ticks: You need to improve your overall attitude and your performance to be able to deal effectively with complainers. You will need to pinpoint the areas needing attention as you go through this module.
- Under 4: A lot of work needs to be done on your skills in dealing with complaints. This chapter will help you identify the areas that most urgently require attention and, with practice, you will improve.

Don't be discouraged if you have a low score. So long as you are keen to improve, you will soon learn the skills you need. Experience is a very important factor when dealing with complaints. Put the work in this chapter into practice, build on your own experience, and you will soon see the results and gain confidence.

Write down any particular areas you need to build confidence in, using the checklist in Figure 7.1.

■

■

■

■

TURN COMPLAINTS INTO OPPORTUNITIES

When you think of the word complaint, what do you think of? Jot down in the space below any words or phrases that occur to you.

Complaints are:

■

■

■

■

The chances are that you have listed mainly negative words. However, there is a positive way of looking at complaints. In fact, looking positively at complaints is the first step on the way to dealing positively with them.

Can you think of any reasons why, or situations where, complaints can be helpful? Jot down anything you can think of below.

■

■

■

■

When a complainer has received a satisfactory response they will tell five or more other people and will talk about it positively.

Every point of contact, every 'moment of truth' with a client is a chance to impress that client, build the relationship and encourage them to return. A complaint is itself another 'moment of truth' and one that can be used very effectively.

A practice needs to welcome complaints as a second chance to keep a client.

Research on complaints, carried out by British Airways, has revealed that customers whose complaints were dealt with efficiently and politely felt even more positive about the airline than they did when everything was right in the first place. Even a complaint made but not satisfactorily dealt with makes the client 10% more likely to come back – just being able to complain helps.

This is not to say that you have to make mistakes just so that you can put them right, of course! It does suggest, though, that you have an excellent opportunity to give your client a little more than they expect when you do put it right.

This is a positive way of looking at complaints.

GENERAL GUIDELINES FOR HANDLING COMPLAINTS

In this section you will put yourself in the client's place and analyse the feelings behind the complaint. That is the best starting point. Once you know how the client feels, you can follow the ten-point plan also described in this section for dealing with complaints.

THINK LIKE A CLIENT

It is essential to bear in mind the attitude and feelings of the client when you are dealing with a complaint. The best way of doing this is to put yourself in the client's shoes.

Have you ever had to take something back to a store to complain about something that you have bought because it was faulty? If you have, take yourself back to the experience for the next activity and remember how it felt. Your reaction typically has three main stages:

- Stage 1: How did you feel when you discovered the fault?
- Stage 2: How did you feel as you decided to take it back?
- Stage 3: How did you feel as you did so? Did you have to brace yourself when you approached the salesperson, for instance?

Typically, you will have a three stage reaction:

- Stage 1: Irritation, frustration at not being able to use the item straight away.
- Stage 2: Annoyance at having to waste time taking it back – wondering whether you should or not, whether you can make time for it or whether it is worth it at all.
- Stage 3: You may have to feel brave to go through with it, so you might have to work to summon up your courage or do it while you still feel angry. (People often feel unsure of themselves when they complain and this can make them more aggressive, as well as extra sensitive to the response they receive.)

So, you could be dealing with someone who is angry or annoyed, rude or aggressive when you deal with a complaint. You could also be dealing with someone who feels uncertain of themselves, who will very easily be put off if your response is rude or off-hand.

To handle an angry client: solve the problem without blaming yourself or anybody else.

SHOW YOU ARE LISTENING TO THE COMPLAINT

There are six levels of listening with increasing degree of attention to the information as follows:

1. Glazed eyes – we've heard nothing!
2. Auto response – something akin to 'yeah, wodevah'!

3. Repeating the last few words – our ability to retrieve using our internal tape recorder.
4. Can ask questions on the information – relevant to what we've just heard, of course.
5. Can tell someone else the information – the minimum we need when listening to complaints.
6. Able to teach someone else – i.e. comfortable answering questions on the information.

If listening is such an everyday activity, why don't we listen? There are many reasons not least because we have been trained to *not* listen – teachers and parents encourage us not to be distracted by something else and listen to them. Among the other reasons why we don't listen might include:

- No interest – the subject or the speaker is just plain boring!
- Distraction – something else is louder or more interesting
- Self talk – our internal dialogue: 'Oh, no... here she goes again... whinge, whinge, whinge...!'
- Delivery of message – voice patterns or volume: 'don't you shout at me!'
- Mismatched body language – 'they don't look angry, they are having a laugh!'
- Waiting to speak – our 'Vickie Pollard Syndrome': anyway-but-no-but-yeah-but-innit?
- Habit pattern – usually from parents who didn't listen to us!
- Defence mechanism – where we delete messages, especially criticism
- Miss the message – due to an emotionally charged distraction (anger/fear/tears!).

When a client complains to you in person or by phone, the most important thing is to make sure they feel you are *really* listening. If you can take the time and space to listen properly first time around, it may well save a lot of extra time and trouble later on!

Ten smart things to do to show you are listening can be found in Figure 7.2.

APOLOGIZE – BUT HOW AND WHAT FOR?

Conventional wisdom suggests that when a client complains, you must apologize at once, whether it is your fault or not. Now, the Veterinary Defence Society (one of the major providers of veterinary indemnity insurance in the UK) suggests that the majority of complaints that it has to deal with are through the client misunderstanding what they have been told – a breakdown in communication. So, rather then apologize for the problem – which may mean you take some degree of liability on behalf of the practice (which your employer would not want you to do) – you can always apologize for the *inconvenience*.

Given that a client can be bothered to complain, and may have had to pluck up courage to confront someone, they will always have felt inconvenienced by

Figure 7.2   Ten smart things to do to show you are listening

Do you:	✓
1. Stay calm and look at them – make eye contact from time to time	☐
2. Apologize for their inconvenience (of having to phone or visit the practice see later)	☐
3. Take the client to a private, seated area or transfer their call to a quiet zone	☐
4. Thank the client for bringing the matter to your attention	☐
5. Ask them to tell you the full story from the beginning	☐
6. Just listen and keep listening – don't interrupt or argue	☐
7. Empathize – but it is generally better to avoid phrases such as 'I know how you feel' (you can't)	☐
8. Pick up on key words, e.g. 'You must have been very worried about X (pet's name)'	☐
9. Take notes and check the client agrees with what you've written	☐
10. Summarize for the client what has been said to ensure you haven't misunderstood or missed anything	☐

having to find your number and dial or actually return to the practice – a special trip for the majority of clients given that they would not have been passing nor live next door!

You are not taking the blame by doing this, but simply apologizing for what has *apparently* happened to inconvenience the client on behalf of the practice. It is a waste of time saying 'I wasn't here at the time' or 'I don't know anything about this'. Passing the buck only makes the situation worse. The client sees you as a representative of the practice and so you must live up to their expectations.

In fact, you probably were not there. Perhaps the client does need to speak to someone else, but if you apologize immediately for their inconvenience, they are more likely to stay calm and feel able to put their complaint reasonably.

- Listen and sympathize; explain what you will do to solve the problem. You can then find the right person to deal with it.
- Keep your cool: be polite and reassuring – and whatever you do don't argue!
- If you can keep your head when your customers are losing theirs and blaming it on you – then you will be a professional!

ON BEING GENUINE

Once you've listened carefully, express regret that the client is dissatisfied; again, apologize for the inconvenience. This is often all the client needs, but it must sound genuine. So, there is no substitute for actually being genuine. More than this:

- Be sincere – the person you're talking to will notice and dislike an automatic response
- Remember, an expression of regret – particularly for the inconvenience – will make the client feel heard and understood. It doesn't mean you are admitting liability – it simply means you are acknowledging the upset and are 'sorry that something has happened', not necessarily 'admitting that it was caused by anyone's fault'.
- Try not to make apologies on behalf of someone else and leave it at that – or let someone else apologize for you. While the individual might not be there to face the client, always get the person involved to follow it up. The client may feel fobbed-off and could end up unhappier than before!
- Get the client on your side by saying things like, 'How can we solve the problem?'

Figure 7.3 is a ten-point plan for dealing with complaints with some gaps – can you fill them in?

(Suggestions are in Figure 7.4 if you need a prompt.)

Summary and suggestions to fill in the gaps of your ten-point plan for dealing with complaints are to be found in Figure 7.4. Why not share these with colleagues to bring them into your practice's working culture?

RESPOND ASSERTIVELY

Situations involving complaints are very often not of your making, as well as unpleasant. However, it is possible to make them more bearable by controlling how you respond. In this section, you will analyse your own behaviour and see the possible consequences of different types of responses.

Figure 7.3 The ten-point plan for dealing with complaints – a draft of five ideas. Can you add the rest?

Do you:
1.
2. Listen carefully: get the facts and details
3.
4. Don't guess at an answer if you don't know it
5.
6. Take action: pass the complaint on to someone else or deal with it yourself
7.
8. Keep calm, polite and provide assurance (that you're willing to help; and prevent a recurrence.)
9.
10. Above all: be professional

Figure 7.4　The complete ten-point plan for dealing with complaints

Do you:
1. Apologize – this is not the same as taking the blame, apologize for the inconvenience that they have been put through
2. Listen carefully: get the facts and details
3. Sympathize: show that you understand the problem. Show that you have heard their complaint
4. Don't guess at an answer if you don't know it
5. Accept responsibility: don't pass the buck. You are not saying that it is your fault. You are apologizing and dealing with the complaint on behalf of the practice
6. Take action: pass the complaint on to someone else or deal with it yourself
7. Tell the client what you are doing: if the process is taking longer than you thought, go back and apologize for the delay. Explain what is happening
8. Keep calm, polite and provide assurance (that you are willing to help; that the problem will not recur)
9. Don't argue: if the client is upsetting you and making you angry, and you can't avoid being dragged into an argument, involve someone else. Quite often, bringing in another person will defuse the situation
10. Above all: be professional

THE 'ABC' RESPONSE PATTERN

The sequence of responses to any situation follows the pattern in Figure 7.5.

In Figure 7.5, you may not be in control of Stage 1, what happens initially, but you can influence Stage 3, the outcome or consequences, by the way you react at Stage 2.

You can respond to an event in three ways.

The aggressive response

You express your feelings and opinions so forcibly that the client is threatened or is made to feel 'small'. An aggressive response can be verbally violent, sarcastic, manipulative or devious. The intention is to get what you want at any cost.

Figure 7.5　The ABC response pattern

The client may go away feeling frustrated, angry or resentful. This client is likely to tell other people about the experience, and their custom will be lost.

A client who has had an unpleasant experience will tell an average of nine or ten other people; 13% of those with a complaint will tell more than 20 others.

The passive response

A passive response can be even more irritating to a client than an aggressive one. This is a response in which the assistant is trying to avoid the issue. She or he might apologize but will not take action and will not reassure the client. The whining tone of voice and feeble body language back up what is being said – often something like 'There's nothing we can do', or 'it's not my fault, it's nothing to do with me'. Customers come away from this experience feeling let down and angry.

The assertive response

Being assertive means being confident, facing up to the issue and trying to find a solution to it. You recognize the client's right to complain and see it as a positive contribution to achieving quality of service. Recognizing your own rights as well as those of the client means you are likely to emerge from the experience feeling that you have done your best and have satisfied the client as far as you could. The client feels reassured and confident that their complaint has been heard and dealt with as well as possible under the circumstances. That is often the most important part of the process.

For smaller purchases such as food items, clothes or household goods, including veterinary products, 37% of unhappy non-complainers will not purchase again; 82% of complainers will if their complaint is handled well.

ASSERTIVENESS STYLE – SELF-TEST

Consider the questions in Figure 7.6 and then tick the box that most clearly describes the frequency with which you display the behaviour.

In Figure 7.6, score your responses according to the following where only your 'always' and 'often' responses are considered.

- If you responded with always or often to questions 1, 2, 7, 9, 14, then you are likely to be adopting a fairly *aggressive* attitude in your working relationships.
- If you responded with always or often to questions 3, 4, 5, 8, 12, 15, 17, then you are likely to be responding to work situations with a fairly *non-assertive* attitude.
- If you responded with always or often to questions 6, 10, 11, 13, 16, then you are likely to be responding to work situations with *assertive* behaviour and communication.

Figure 7.6 The Assertiveness Style – self test. Tick the box that most clearly describes the frequency with which you display the behaviour

Behaviour:	Always	Often	Sometimes	Never
1. I have difficulty dealing calmly with angry people				
2. I find myself becoming quite angry if I feel that people are trying to take advantage of me – and I let them know				
3. When my views or actions are challenged I feel intimidated				
4. Because it is important to me that people hold a good opinion of me, I tend to go along with the majority view				
5. I prefer a peaceful life and don't like to make waves				
6. In difficult situations, I am able to control my emotions and hold my ground				
7. I like to be in control of what's happening				
8. There are some people who have the knack of making me feel inadequate – and I find myself agreeing with them when I would really prefer not to				
9. I can be volatile and quick-tempered when things aren't going my way				
10. I make a real effort to seek a win/win outcome				
11. I consider that what I have to say is equally as important as anything anyone else might have to say				
12. I can say no to colleagues and subordinates, but I find it hard to say no to someone who has power over me				
13. I have the confidence to ask for what I want – even if I might risk upsetting someone else				
14. In business, the end justifies the means and I do whatever I think is necessary				
15. I think good teamwork depends on a harmonious working atmosphere – so I go out of my way to avoid disagreeing with colleagues				
16. I can bite the bullet and say what I think, honestly and directly				
17. When problems occur, I automatically assume responsibility for causing the problem				

THE CONSEQUENCES OF YOUR AGGRESSIVE BEHAVIOUR

These can be long term and potentially quite serious, both for you and everyone around you. They include:

- health problems such as ulcers, hypertension, migraine, exhaustion
- feelings of guilt or regret
- breakdown of communication in the practice
- loss of trust and respect among clients and colleagues
- isolation from colleagues and friends
- short-term and long-term damage to your work resulting from:
  - shortage of information: people are unwilling to confront you with the truth because they know how you are most likely to react
  - shortage of specialist knowledge: you haven't given people a genuine opportunity to contribute to helping you at work
  - limited access to the grapevine – you'll be excluded
- inability to call in 'favours': you don't help anyone, so why should they help you?
- short-term and long-term damage to career prospects.

If you regularly use aggressive behaviour, you may reap short-term rewards, such as getting your own way or achieving power over others. The down side is that people will seek to avoid you and, wherever possible, they will make sure that you are excluded from developmental projects that require a creative and organic approach. Ultimately, people will work against you.

THE CONSEQUENCES OF YOUR NON-ASSERTIVE BEHAVIOUR

These can be equally serious and include:

- health problems, such as depression, lower back pain, digestive problems, insomnia
- feelings of anger, frustration and self-pity
- a downward spiral of low confidence and low self-esteem
- loss of respect
- breakdown of work relationships as people realize that they are able to take advantage of you... and then they feel guilty
- short-term and long-term damage to your work resulting from:
  - missed deadlines: your inability to say no means that you (and your colleagues) take on unrealistic amounts of work and then are unable to complete work on time
  - poor teamwork: your inability to take a firm line with aggressive colleagues may lead to squabbles, arguments, confrontations and, ultimately, a total breakdown of working relationships on the team
  - ill-conceived ideas: because you find yourself unable to control aggressive colleagues you could find yourself held responsible for a client complaining about them as colleagues realize they can be as outrageous and experimental as they like
- short-term and long-term damage to career prospects.

If you regularly use non-assertive behaviour, you may often reap short-term rewards, such as avoiding unpleasantness or keeping everyone happy. The down side is that you will become increasingly frustrated and anxious as people begin to assume that you will agree to their demands. You will feel that you are losing control and that your preferences, opinions and ideas carry little weight with the team.

THE REWARDS OF ASSERTIVE BEHAVIOUR

The benefits include:

- fewer stress-related health problems
- improved self-confidence, self-esteem and self-respect
- increased respect from others
- improved work relationships as people begin to:
  - gain confidence in your honesty and openness
  - realize that you say what you mean, and mean what you say – they recognize that you are a 'safe pair of hands' – they know where they stand
  - feel free to make suggestions and offer up creative ideas – they willingly share information
- short-term and long-term benefits for your work include:
  - improved teamwork: the aggressive people realize that they will not be able to intimidate you, the non-assertive people recognize they will be listened to. Everyone begins to understand that you are prepared to discuss, negotiate and – where necessary – compromise
- short-term and long-term career benefits.

People begin to realize that you have the confidence to voice your opinions and ideas reasonably and calmly. They come to see you as someone who will not be intimidated or manipulated, who will work at creating harmonious relationships and who operates with a high degree of firmness, integrity and honesty.

ASSERTIVE BEHAVIOUR IN ACTION

Being assertive involves operating from a position where you recognize that:

- you have the right to be heard and so does everyone else
- you have the right to hold your own views, opinions and beliefs and so does everyone else
- you have something to contribute and so does everyone else
- you have the right to disagree and to say 'no' and so does everyone else.

The aggressive position is, generally, 'I alone have these rights', while the non-assertive position is 'Everyone has these rights…except me'.

ASSERTIVE COMMUNICATION

Assertive communication consists of three simple steps, which are shown below:

- Step 1: Listen and acknowledge that you have heard and understood the other person's point of view. Ask open questions if you need more information
- Step 2: Express, clearly and calmly, your own position and feelings
- Step 3: Make constructive suggestions about what could or should happen next

The three steps involved in assertive communication are now described in more detail.

Step 1 Demonstrate that you've heard and understood

The first step in the process involves making a clear and simple statement that acknowledges whatever has been said. This is important because, if you are dealing with an aggressive person who feels that what they have said has been ignored or brushed aside, then they will become even more aggressive. Non-assertive people will have great difficulty in repeating their question or request, but will inwardly burn with anger and frustration. This can prove to be an explosive combination that may ignite sometime in the future, when you are least expecting it.

Step 2 Express your own feelings and views

Find out more, if you need to. Be direct and honest, and don't be frightened to use 'I' and 'my' statements like:

- 'I'd like it if...'
- 'I think that...'
- 'I feel...'
- 'In my opinion...'
- 'My view is that...'

Don't jump to conclusions, and be prepared to take the time to find out more. Ask open how? Why? What? When? and Where? questions like:

- How do you think we should deal with this?
- What, in your view, is the main problem?
- What changes would you like to see?
- What would your approach be?

Even if someone's opinions are diametrically opposed to yours, do remember that they have the right to hold their own opinions. But also remember that being assertive is about maintaining your own position, even when someone is being aggressive and pushing you hard.

Step 3 Make constructive suggestions as to what might happen next

Often it's not enough just to say 'No' or 'That's not what I want'. Be prepared to make suggestions or offer alternatives. For example:

- 'My view is that we have to proceed very carefully with this, but we could think about…'
- 'I feel that right now would be the wrong time to change client records. Even so, I recognize your concern, and it would be helpful to know if you think there is another time, later this year, when we could introduce these new ideas.'
- 'I'm very concerned that you have not been able to meet the deadline we agreed. The key step we need to take now is to create a plan to finish the job by the weekend – What do you suggest?'

CORE STATEMENTS

Working out your core statement can be a very useful exercise when you know, in advance, that you have to:

- confront someone and explain your dissatisfaction
- stand firm to your point of view in the face of strong opposition
- ask for something you want
- refuse a request.

To create a core statement, simply focus on your objective. Think about what you want to achieve as a result of the communication. Here are some examples of core statements which match the list given above.

- Confront someone and explain your dissatisfaction
  - 'I'm extremely concerned by the client being told they need not pay their bill when I'd insisted they pay like everyone else; this undermines my position as receptionist and I can't be expected to deal with clients effectively for the practice.'
  - 'I feel that the way you spoke to the new receptionist was inappropriate and you hurt her feelings. I would like you to, please, not take your anger out on youngsters so that we can all work together for the common interests of maintaining animal welfare.'
  - 'I am very sorry that the information you received was not as clear as it might have been and that you have been inconvenienced by the problem. I will be happy to discuss the best solution for you if you'd like to meet with the practice manager in her office.'
- Stand firm to your point of view in the face of strong opposition
  - 'I understand your concerns, but I am convinced, having seen the meeting report, that we have no alternative but to wait until next year.'
  - 'I can see this is important to you but, in my opinion, the plan won't work because there isn't enough in the budget to cover all the additional costs.'
  - 'I can see why you think we ought to wait but, in my opinion, if we're going to do this, we need to do it now before we lose our competitive edge.'

- Ask for something you want
  - 'I recognize that money is tight, but I really need another member of staff if we're to improve service at reception over the busy periods.'
  - 'I know there have been difficulties in the past, but I really need to spend some time on the client records, if I'm going to find a solution to the problem.'
  - 'I can see why you don't want another delay but, in my opinion, we must wait until the new receptionist is properly familiar with procedures before we leave her unsupervised at the branch practice.'

Your core statement should be your bottom line, ideal outcome. Of course, as part of the process of searching for a win/win outcome you may have to negotiate and, to some extent, compromise. But, at the very least, if you give your core statement some serious thought before the encounter, you will have a clear idea of what you want the outcome to be.

SAYING 'NO!'

Many people have great difficulty with refusing requests and saying 'No!' An aggressive refusal to a reasonable request can cause terrific resentment: 'I only asked if I could move my car and she went ballistic!' A non-assertive refusal can leave the petitioner wondering whether the answer was yes or no: 'I went in, asked if I could change the schedules, he rambled on for nearly twenty minutes and I've come out of his office and I still don't know. What a waste of time!'

People often mistakenly believe that if they say no, people will:

- get angry and cause a scene
- feel resentful and, at a later date, take some kind of revenge
- spread gossip and rumour about the refusal
- perceive the person saying 'no' in a very negative way.

Robyn, a veterinary receptionist, explains:

> 'I just hate having to say 'No'. I always feel guilty; and I always think that people will feel angry or let down if I refuse a request. So I can never really win. If I say 'No', I feel guilty or anxious…and I always seem to spend ages apologizing. If I say 'Yes', I often feel irritated or frustrated because, afterwards, I wish I'd had the courage to say 'No'. It's hopeless.'

If you are caught in a similar spiral, the key points to remember are:

- When you say 'No', you are merely refusing the request and not rejecting the person.
- Refusals can be simple, open and honest statements.

Let us review five ways of saying 'no'.

Not now, but then

This is useful when you cannot do something immediately, yet you leave the person in no doubt that you are willing to help:

- 'No, I can't do the cleaning now but I will do it when I have made these calls to clients.'
- 'No, I can't do that today, but I can do it tomorrow when the vaccine reminders have gone out.'

No, with a reason

If you feel it is appropriate, you can soften your refusal by giving a reason for saying no:

- 'No, I can't work at the weekend *because* I'm helping my family get Granny into her flat.'
- 'No, I can't let you have a repeat prescription *because* this product has restrictions on its use.'

No, with an alternative

Offering an alternative is another technique you can use when you feel that a straightforward no might be inappropriate, for example when dealing with an important client or a very senior colleague.

- 'No, I can't promise that I'll be able to get her in today. I can, however, assure you that I can get her in by the 22nd July.'
- 'No, I don't feel that that approach would get the results we need. What I would like to suggest is that we talk to the practice manager before we make a decision.'

Simple no

Sometimes a simple, straightforward no is all that is required. Don't apologize and don't beat around the bush. Just calmly and clearly say 'No'.

- 'No. I'm not prepared to mislead anyone on the facts.'
- 'No. I'm not willing to agree to that.'

Broken record no

The broken record is a useful technique when you find yourself dealing with manipulative or aggressive people who will simply not take no for an answer. In some situations, you will find it useful to work out what your core statement is before you get involved in the conversation. Imagine a conversation as follows:

You: 'No, I can't promise that I'll be able to get her in today. I can, however, assure you that I can take her in on the 22ⁿᵈ.'

Client:' But you've never let me down before!'

You: 'And I don't intend to let you down this time. I can't promise that I'll be able to get her in today because the operation was cancelled and we are now full. I can promise that I can take her in on the 22ⁿᵈ.'

Client: 'But surely, if you pull out all the stops, get extra people in...'

You: 'Because the operation was cancelled, we cannot do it today at short notice. If we had stayed with the original booking, I could have had her in today in time to meet your deadline. But now I can't promise to do that. I can take her in on the 22ⁿᵈ.'

Client: 'But you said you could have it done by the 19ᵗʰ.'

You: 'Yes, you're right. And that is what we originally agreed. Your husband cancelled that date and I can't get her in today, the 19ᵗʰ, which was the original booking. I can assure you that I can book her in, now that you want to go ahead, by the 22ⁿᵈ.'

The key points to remember, when using the broken record technique, are to keep your nerve and continue to repeat your core statement.

YOUR RIGHTS

As we have already mentioned, everyone (that means you and the rest of the world) has certain rights. These are shown below and you may find it helpful, as part of your assertiveness strategy, to photocopy the list and keep it beside your desk as a constant reminder. As an alternative, discuss the list with your colleagues and agree a format for your practice – it would be good to get the Partners involved, too!

YOU HAVE THE RIGHT TO:

say No

express your views, opinions and beliefs (even if they are different from the mainstream)

ask for what you want (while recognizing that you might not always get it!)

change your mind (in the light of new information or circumstances)

make mistakes (because everyone does)

not know or understand (because you can't be expected to know and understand everything)

make your own choices (because you know what you need and what suits you best)

be yourself (without compromising others)

SECTION SUMMARY

To be able to deal with client complaints positively, you need to:

- put yourself in the client's place
- listen to the complaint sympathetically
- respond assertively and appropriately and take action – whether that means dealing with the problem yourself, finding someone who can or suggesting alternatives.

KEY TIPS

PROFIT FROM COMPLAINTS

- A complaint is a second chance to get it right.
- Turn complaints into opportunities.
- Deal positively and professionally with a complaint.
- Think like a client.
- Solve the problem without blaming yourself or anyone else.

The ten-point plan

1. Apologize
2. Listen
3. Sympathize
4. Don't guess at an answer if you don't know
5. Accept responsibility on behalf of the practice
6. Take action
7. Explain what you are doing
8. Keep calm, provide assurance
9. Don't argue
10. Be professional

HANDLING COMPLAINTS: DOS AND DON'TS

Do

- Listen
- Sympathize
- Ask questions
- Take control firmly
- Suggest a course of action
- Gain agreement to it
- Follow the action through.

Don't

- Overreact
- Become agitated

- Become defensive
- Feel guilty
- Pretend to know things
- Make promises you cannot keep.

HANDLING SPECIFIC TYPES OF PEOPLE

Angry

- Don't get angry in return.
- Don't try being terribly logical, it'll make matters worse.
- Don't agree with sweeping statements. Think first.
- Don't make excuses about other staff, busy, new, etc.
- Do apologize for specific items, as appropriate.
- Do suggest ways of putting the matter right.

Whingeing

- Never show you're bored or frustrated.
- Do continue to look interested.
- Don't bully or try to dominate, or interrupt rudely.
- Do take advantage of every pause for breath.
- Get back to facts.
- Get the direction you want to go.

The rude

- Do remain cool and professionally detached.
- Do stay polite at all times.
- Do make repeated offers of specific action that'll help.
- Don't go all icy and withdrawn.
- Don't make smart remarks and try to score points.
- Don't be driven into an emotional response.
- Don't take it personally. Try to ignore the rudeness.

The suspicious

- Don't become irritated by persistent questioning.
- Don't allow checking and re-checking to upset you.
- Never make vague statements, stick to facts.
- Don't make statements you are not certain about, you'll be caught out.

The know-it-all

- Don't pretend to know things that you don't.
- Don't pour scorn on mistakes that you hear. You might be right, but you won't win.

- Don't plead ignorance without explaining that you will fetch someone who does know.
- Do appear impressed by correct knowledge and, if necessary, tend to flatter, if it allows you to make your own points.

Silence

- Don't give up!
- Do ask open questions to establish what is wrong.
- Do be reassuring.

Now you have read this chapter, add some ideas for action to your list in the Appendix.

Chapter 8
Client service solutions

In this chapter, we look at the variety of reasons why people have problems and what we can do to improve matters – or at the very least, not make it any worse. (The approach we take in this chapter is presented as a workbook inviting you to consider your approach, jot your answers in a space provided, and then look at some suggestions.) From problems, we turn to explore strategies and tactics to show our willingness to solve the problems and lead to a successful conclusion. But first, a fundamental question:

WHY DO CLIENTS HAVE PROBLEMS?

Clients have all kinds of problems, and these are usually because:

- They are unable to get the product or the service they want.
- They are unhappy about the quality of the product or service they have purchased.
- They have been inconvenienced by the systems, procedures and/or 'red tape' of the practice where they bought (or are trying to buy) a product or service.
- Someone has upset them in the practice, either because someone has been rude or bad-tempered, or because someone has been careless or made a mistake.

The way in which a client complains will depend on a number of factors including:

- What kind of person they are.
- How upset they are by the problem.
- Whether this is the first time they have had to complain about the problem, or whether they have complained before.

Some clients may make a great deal of fuss over what may appear to be a trivial problem. From a client service point of view, it is really important to recognize that a problem, which may seem insignificant to you, may be very important to the client. It is important to recognize that every client problem, no matter how small or insignificant it may appear to you, should be treated with equal care and attention. This is because:

- Small problems that are not handled properly may quickly grow into big problems that can cause considerable distress for the client. The end result may mean major disruption or even expense when the practice has to rectify the small problem that has grown into a major disaster.

Every client problem (whether large or small), which is not dealt with efficiently, may result in a lost client. No business can afford to lose clients and it is worth remembering that the client who spends £2 today may well be someone who plans to spend £200 tomorrow.

A problem that seems insignificant or unimportant to you may be perceived by the client as extremely important!

Good client service is vital for the survival of any business, regardless of whether it is a large, mixed, or small animal practice. The same is true of your local restaurants, hairdressers, clothes shops, food stores, and opticians and, in fact, any business that relies on making sales to the general public.

Because of the increased choice available to them, clients can pick and choose where they want to spend their money. For instance, if they don't like what is on offer at Practice 'A', then they can go to Practice 'B' and get the same product, an operation, or advice. If they think Practice 'A's prices are too high, relative to what they get for their money, or the client service is poor, then they will spend their money with Practice 'B'.

Practices that offer the best choice and value for the price, together with the best client service, will both keep their old clients and persuade new clients to do business with them. This means, of course, that the business will stay open and continue to trade and so can be sure of providing job security for the staff.

Dealing sensitively with client problems is an extremely important part of providing good client care and goes a long way towards ensuring that clients continue to spend money with a business.

No doubt, as a customer yourself, you have made numerous complaints over the years regarding various products and services. The complaints you have made may have been to do with faulty or damaged goods, or delivery delays, errors, mistakes and mix-ups or unprofessional behaviour from staff. No matter what your experience was, you will probably not be willing to spend money again with a business that in the past provided poor client service. In fact, why should you? And you most probably mentioned the experience to someone else you know, either at home or at work. Perhaps hearing about your problems may have persuaded them to shop elsewhere in the future, so creating a ripple effect which has resulted in a fair amount of lost business for the business concerned.

On the other hand, though, if you have dealt with an organization where your problem or complaint has been dealt with courteously, helpfully and efficiently, and you were made to feel like a valued and appreciated client, then you will probably be happy to continue to give them your business in the future.

CHECKLIST

Providing excellent client service involves always:

treating clients with courtesy and efficiency

treating clients as individuals with individual needs

putting clients first, rather than routines, systems or procedures

making clients feel valued

giving each and every problem (no matter how small or insignificant it may appear to you) equal care and attention

making the client the most important person to you at that moment when you are dealing with them

UNDERSTANDING THE PROBLEM

Before you can start to solve your client's problem you must, of course, be absolutely clear about the nature of the problem. Some clients are able to explain concisely exactly what is wrong, while other clients may give a confusing or rambling description. Some people may be so angry or upset that it can be very difficult to get a clear picture.

Your first task when dealing with a client problem is to identify exactly what is wrong and why the client is unhappy. Until you do this, you will not be in a position to help.

ACTIVITY 1

What are the two most important skills you need to use when identifying the nature of a client's problem?

1.

2.

What are the four key pieces of information you need to know about the problem?

1.

2.

3.

4.

(You are invited to consider your approach, jot your answers in the space provided, and then continue reading the text to look at some suggestions)

The two most important skills you need to use when identifying the nature of a problem are the skills of:

■ listening and
■ questioning

Because you will only be able to find out the real nature of the problem by listening carefully to what the client has to say and by asking appropriate questions to obtain all the relevant information you need. We will be looking at this in detail further on in this section.

When you are dealing with any kind of client problem the key pieces of information you need to gather from the client are:

1. What does he or she think the problem is?
   Sometimes, the client's perception of the problem may be quite different to yours. Take the situation where a client complains that a flea spray that she bought from you for her cat did not kill the fleas and it made the cat's coat dull, losing its shine. Now which is the major problem? You might be forgiven for thinking that her distress was caused by both these factors. In fact, she might not mind the product not working immediately – thinking it only a transitory thing while the spray took hold of the flea problem – but that the coat condition being affected ruined the cat's chances at the children's school pet show was the real issue! That would be the heart of the matter.
2. What is the history of the problem?
   When did the problem occur?
   Has the client complained about this specific problem before?
   What, if anything, has already been done so far to rectify the problem?
3. What is the current situation?
   What is happening right now?
   What is wrong with the product or service?
   Where is the product?
   What condition is the product in?
4. What does the client want?
   What, for the client, would be the ideal solution?

(Remember that their ideal solution may be different to yours. For instance, you might think that they want a refund when, in fact, they want a replacement.)

Clearly, you will only be able to obtain all this information by careful listening and questioning.

UNDERSTANDING, ACKNOWLEDGING AND OWNING PROBLEMS

In addition to asking questions and listening carefully, it is equally important that you let the client know that you acknowledge and own the problem.

CASE STUDY

During her lunch hour, Pauline bought a medicated cat-collar from a large mixed practice in the centre of her local town where she worked. That evening, she put the elasticated flea collar on the cat according to the instructions given to her – then she washed her hands as advised. The next time she saw her cat, the following evening, she noticed the cat was not steady on its legs and seemed quite listless. She took the collar off immediately and kept an eye on her cat. The next morning the cat seemed fine, but it was not for a couple of days that Pauline could get away at lunch, but she returned to the practice with the collar and spoke to the receptionist. She explained what had happened and then the conversation went like this:

Pauline: *So what are you going to do about it?*
Receptionist: Perhaps it was something the cat picked up and ate.
Pauline: *She is a house cat and I haven't changed her food.*
Receptionist: Must be its food.
Pauline: *I said I haven't changed her food! Look, I don't think you understand what I'm saying.*
Receptionist: Well anyway, I'll need to talk to Sylvia the nurse, and she's on her lunch.
Pauline: *Yes, so am I, but what are you going to do about it.*
Receptionist: Well, as I said, I'll need to talk to Sylvia. Can you come back after lunch?
Pauline: *No I can't! I'm in a hurry.*
Receptionist: Well I'm sorry, I can't do anything until I've spoken to Sylvia and she won't be back from lunch until gone 2 o'clock, knowing her.

Imagine that you have to deal with Pauline and her problem.

Activity 2
What would you have said in order to show that you:

1. Understand the problem
2. Acknowledge the problem
3. Own the problem

UNDERSTANDING THE PROBLEM

The best way to show someone that you understand what they have said is to summarize the key points of their conversation. For example:

So you noticed that your cat, Moggie, was a little listless after she had worn the collar for a day or so.

Summarizing gives the client the opportunity to correct any misunderstandings.

Yes, and she was not walking well.

ACKNOWLEDGING THE PROBLEM

This involves showing the client that you recognize there is a problem and accepting that they have some emotional feelings about the issue, i.e. that they are upset, angry, inconvenienced or whatever. It is the difference between:

'Oh, I see!' and

'You must have been really upset when you saw Moggie behaving like that.'

Remember, it is tempting to get on with solving the problem for the client but, until they feel that you are 'on their side', in other words, with them rather than against them, they may not listen to you. How many times have you felt that they 'wanted to speak to someone in authority' and you were 'just' the receptionist? (The author has met thousands of veterinary receptionists while delivering training courses and at the BVNA/BSAVA/VPMA congresses and has not yet met any one called 'Just'!)

Our friends, people we turn to to chat about our woes, are very good (usually) at listening and *validating* our emotions. By this is meant that they empathize and sympathize with us.

Empathy is when someone 'knows how you feel', they have shared the experience.

Sympathy is when someone 'feels sorry for you' having to 'put-up with that'.

Note: you *cannot* 'empathize' with someone suffering something as personal as bereavement, but you could, for example, empathize with someone who feels cross that they were misinformed:

You might say, for example, 'Oh how annoying for you – I'd feel cross if I had been told the wrong thing'.

In this way, while you can *apologize* for the feelings they have... 'I am very sorry for the trouble you have taken to come back into the practice...', you do not have to make an admission of guilt on something that may need a more senior person to deal with or where you are not yet sure of all the facts.

So, by acknowledging the effect the problem has had on the individual, without being patronizing, they may calm down a little so that you can get more information to help you understand the problem a little deeper. This may help you to find better solutions, too.

OWNING THE PROBLEM

Owning the problem involves accepting responsibility for putting it right and not attempting to pass the buck to someone else. It is the difference between:

'Well, I'll have to talk to the person who served you' and

'Well, first of all let me apologize for the inconvenience and worry you've had and let me see what I can do to sort it out for you.'

The key point here is that when clients have a problem they are not interested in anything but getting their problems solved and having their difficulties sorted out as quickly, easily and smoothly as possible.

Obviously, you should never make promises you cannot keep and, of course, every business has its own systems and procedures for dealing with client returns, complaints and so on. Nevertheless, it is important to show clients that you understand, acknowledge and own the problem and that you will, as far as you are able, sort it out for them.

Clients who feel that they have not been listened to and that their problem has not been properly understood will get angry. Clients get very angry when they are made to feel that the person listening to their problem does not really acknowledge it and is trying to shift responsibility for solving it onto someone else.

DEALING WITH DIFFICULT CLIENTS

Clients come in all shapes, sizes, moods and tempers. Sometimes clients are pleasant, well spoken, smartly dressed people who are a pleasure to deal with. Sometimes, though, clients can be described, at best, as difficult.

The key to providing consistent, meaningful client service is to ensure that all your clients are treated with equal care, courtesy and consideration, no matter how difficult their behaviour might be.

ACTIVITY 3

Imagine that you are doing your absolute best to deal courteously and efficiently with your client but, no matter what approach you take, she responds by being grumpy, irritable, sarcastic, bad-tempered and down-right difficult. List four possible reasons for your client's bad behaviour.

1.

2.

3.

4.

(Remember, you are invited to consider your approach, jot your answers in the space provided, and then continue reading the text to look at some suggestions)

Clients can, from time to time, behave badly and it is important to recognize that there is always a reason for this behaviour and this may, or may not, be something to do with you.

Reasons that have nothing to do with you include:

1. The client is feeling ill
   This could be anything from a minor illness like a headache or backache that is painful, right through to something very serious and severe such as cancer.
2. The client is feeling worried
   Something fairly minor like an unexpected bill, or something very serious such as an impending job loss, divorce or house repossession might cause the worry.
3. The client is feeling upset
   Maybe they have just had an argument at work or at home, their partner has just left them, another of their pets has died, the central heating has broken down, the car has been stolen or the roof is leaking.

4. The client is feeling annoyed

Perhaps the last time they dealt with your practice they did not receive good client service, or perhaps the product they bought did not live up to their expectations, maybe one of your vets was short with them, or maybe someone in a shop or garage has just been rude to them.

The key point to remember is that in all of these cases, the client will not tell you the reason why they are feeling ill or worried or upset or annoyed. The important thing is not to take the client's behaviour personally. Remain calm, friendly, courteous and professional while you are attempting to solve their problem.

Concentrate on:

- obtaining the information
- understanding the problem
- acknowledging there is a problem – validate the emotion
- owning the problem
- reassuring the client that whatever can be done, will be done.

Clients may also behave badly in response to the behaviour that is shown to them. This works on the basis of:

If you are going to be rude to me, then I'm going to be rude to you.

Clients who have a genuine problem and who sometimes begin by presenting their complaint calmly and politely, can end the conversation in a very different frame of mind. This change of attitude is almost always due to the behaviour and attitude of the person with whom they are dealing.

The next activity will give you an opportunity to think about the sorts of thing you might do, when dealing with a client problem, which could upset and annoy the client and make matters worse than they already are.

ACTIVITY 4

List four things you might do, either on purpose or by accident, which might upset, irritate or annoy a client when you are attempting to solve their problem or deal with a complaint.

1.

2.

3.

4.

Clients can be upset by:

- Use of slang: words like dear (particularly upsetting for many women clients), love, mate, sunshine, flower, pet and so on should never be used by professionals in a professional situation.

- Carrying on another conversation at the same time: when you are dealing with a client problem, the client should have your full and undivided attention for as long as it takes.
- Arguing, contradicting or suggesting that the client is being less than truthful: of course there may be times when you have good reason to believe that the client is not being totally truthful, but arguing or contradicting will only make matters worse. Use tact and diplomacy to deal with every client problem and allow the documentation (case notes, appointment books, invoices, receipts, and so on) to speak for themselves.
- Judging on appearance: do not make assumptions about clients solely based on their appearance. Just because someone is not smartly dressed, it does not mean that they should be treated as anything other than a valued client.
- Making promises that can't be kept: always be totally truthful and honest in your dealings with clients. For instance, if the delivery date of a replacement item is likely to be three weeks rather than two, say so. Nothing is more irritating, from a client's point of view, than being made promises or assurances that are unrealistic or untrue.
- Showing favouritism: all clients deserve equal care and attention. Paying more attention to clients who are more attractive, or who are regular clients or who seem as though they are ready to make a fuss will upset other, equally important, clients.
- Criticizing your practice or your colleagues: clients do not want to hear your criticisms of how other people have dealt with the problem so far, nor do they want to hear your negative views about the practice you work for. Criticizing others is both disloyal and unprofessional.

HANDLING INFORMATION

Some client problems are fairly straightforward in that the client presents the information verbally (tells you what has happened) and you have sufficient data to enable you to sort out the situation straight away. Other problems can be more complex because, from a client service point of view, you need information from a number of different sources, as well as from the client.

Sometimes this may be written information, for example:

- receipt
- invoice
- pre-op' advice
- post-op' advice
- purchase order – of orders you place on behalf of a client
- delivery note – of material delivered to the practice.

Sometimes it may be verbal information from other people such as colleagues within your practice, or manufacturers or suppliers from outside the practice. The information provided by people may be:

- explanations
- confirmations
- facts and/or figures.

When gathering information relating to a client problem it is very important that you:

- check the accuracy of the information. (When did you sell them the product, when did they collect the animal, when was it ordered, how did they pay? Have they paid?)
- take into account whether the person (or people) supplying the information has a vested interest. (If the client's mother confirms the client's perception of the problem, does the client's mother have a vested interest?)

All the information gathered could be described as either quantitative or qualitative:

Quantitative – which relates to measurable facts:

- I waited 3 days
- I paid £17.50
- I telephoned 4 times.

Qualitative – which relates to feelings and perceptions about the problem:

- I'm very angry with this…
- I've been passed from one person to another…
- I was told that…

Gathering, sifting, analysing and recording all of the information is a vital part of identifying and dealing with client problems. It is necessary to gather the information so that you have a complete picture of the client's problem, and it is necessary to record the information accurately so that all of the facts relating to the problem can be passed on to someone else or are on file for the future in case:

- someone else in the practice needs to access the information
- the problem recurs
- there is a query from the manufacturer or supplier.

All written information relating to a client's problem should be:

- neat and legible
- clearly labelled with your name, the client's name and other details, and the date
- give a clear and concise summary of:
    - the nature of the problem
    - the action which was taken to deal with the problem
- separate pieces of paper should be securely clipped together, or stored in a folder so that nothing gets lost!

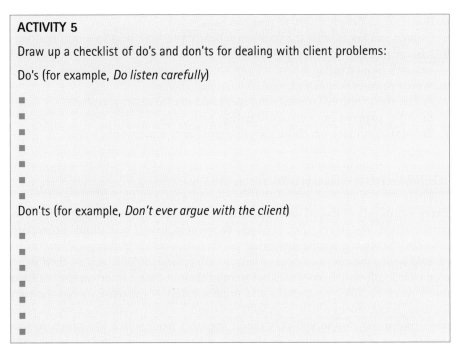

ACTIVITY 5

Draw up a checklist of do's and don'ts for dealing with client problems:

Do's (for example, *Do listen carefully*)

-
-
-
-
-
-
-

Don'ts (for example, *Don't ever argue with the client*)

-
-
-
-
-
-
-

Your checklist for dealing with client problems might include:

Do:

- Listen carefully and concentrate on what is being said.
- Summarize what has been said to give the client an opportunity to correct any misunderstandings.
- Use open and encouraging body language – nodding, smiling, maintaining good eye contact.
- Ask open questions to obtain all the information.
- Take notes if the problem is complex.
- Allow the client to 'let off steam' if they need to.
- Show the client that you understand, acknowledge and own the problem.
- Reassure the client that you will do everything possible to resolve the problem.
- Find out what the client wants.
- Explain what you propose to do to solve the problem, and obtain agreement to your chosen course of action.
- Keep the client informed and up-to-date if there are any delays or unexpected hitches.

Don't:

- Argue, interrupt or talk-over the client.
- Show that you are irritable or angry.
- Ask leading questions.

- Blame other people or try to pass the buck.
- Assume you know what the problem is before you have heard the whole story.
- Assume you know what the client wants you to do until you have checked this out with him or her.
- Make promises you can't keep.
- Be less than truthful to pacify the client and get them off your back.
- Rush the paperwork or the information gathering.
- Say or do anything which might cause the client unnecessary worry.

GENERATING SOLUTIONS

Every organization has its own procedures and systems for dealing with client complaints. Some stores, such as Marks & Spencer, have a very simple procedure whereby clients can return unwanted goods and, providing the goods are fit to be sold again, the client can either have a cash refund, a debit against their store credit card, gift vouchers or another item of their choice. Other companies have much more complex procedures and require proof of purchase within the past 28 days. Some stores refuse to refund cash and are only willing to issue a credit note, and so on. Some will only credit the card from which the purchase was made – even if it is presented by the wife of the purchaser using the same joint account!

Obviously, it is extremely important that you understand the procedures that your practice uses to resolve client complaints.

ACTIVITY 6

What kind of information should be covered in a practice's complaints procedures?

For example: 'What to do if...'

the client damages or misuses a product and then asks for a replacement.

a client returns an item that is only part used, like a carton of kitten milk-replacer.

List five key pieces of information that should be contained in a complaints procedure. (Perhaps ask some colleagues in the practice for some ideas.) So, *our complaints procedure should contain what to do if:*

1.

2.

3.

4.

5.

The information that is most usually contained in complaints procedures includes what to do if:

- a retail product is faulty (is broken, does not do what it is supposed to do, etc.)
- the product has been damaged or misused by the client (has been broken, used incorrectly, etc.)
- the service from the practice has not met client expectations
- veterinary or nursing or reception staff have not met client expectations
- the product is part used
- the bill is more than expected
- the product must be repaired or replaced by the manufacturer and should also give details of the circumstances under which a refund, a replacement, no refund or replacement can be made.

Generally, client complaints relate to:

- product/service faults
- bill/account/paperwork faults
- ordering faults
- delivery faults
- staff attitude or behaviour faults.

An effective and efficient organization should have a procedure to deal with each of these types of complaints.

ASKING FOR HELP

Some client problems are very straightforward and can be dealt with quickly and easily without reference to anyone else. Take, for instance, a situation where a client returns a flea collar in perfect condition, in its unopened original packing together with the appropriate receipt and asks for a simple exchange for another size or colour. This is the kind of problem that can be dealt with straight away. Other problems are much more demanding and complex and require the attention of more than one person within the practice.

There could be a number of occasions when you might need help or advice from someone else, and these include situations where:

- You do not have access to information.
- The problem is completely new or very complicated, and you do not have the experience or expertise to solve it.
- You do not have the authority.
- You have decided on the best solution, but you need to check with someone else that your solution is acceptable or possible.
- The solution you have presented to the client is unacceptable to them and you need to find an alternative.
- The client is extremely irate and out of control and you need help to calm them down.

In any of these situations you may need to ask for help or advice from:

- a colleague
- a veterinary nurse
- the practice manager
- a veterinary surgeon
- one of the partners
- (perhaps via someone else) but to the manufacturer of a product
- a supplier of a service – like a laboratory, again maybe through someone else.

It is very important that you:

- are prepared to ask other people for information, help and advice if and when you need it
- know whom to ask.

COOPERATION TECHNIQUES

This section gives you a few useful techniques to help you deal with complaints.

Technique 1: solve the problem

Think of 'How to solve the problem' rather than 'Who is to blame'?
Even if you do not say so to the client, sometimes it is easy to think:

'That's not my job'
or 'Nobody told me…'
or 'That happened when I wasn't here…'
or 'I don't see why I should sort out somebody else's mess…'

And sometimes it is easy to blame yourself when a situation goes wrong. You might think:

'I knew I should have…'
'I've made a real mess of this…'
'I can't get anything right.'

Blaming either yourself or other people is a waste of time. This is not to say that you can't recognize a mistake and learn from it. However, using your energy trying to find out who is to blame just makes you feel angry, resentful or sorry for yourself. It achieves nothing worthwhile. In a job that involves dealing with client complaints, you are almost always sorting out situations that are not directly your fault. The answer is to solve the problem and take it professionally and see it as just another part of your job.

Technique 2: find out what they want you to do

Listen carefully and repeat what the client has said to check you have understood and know what they want you to do.

Often a client will approach you with a complaint and with no suggestions for the solution. He or she might tell you exactly what is wrong. You will be told the whole story and why it caused such problems but often you are left to suggest the solution yourself.

Situation…

You have apologized, listened sympathetically, shown that you understand. What do you do next?

Technique 3: outline the solution, or the alternatives

Handling an angry person with a complaint is quite simple when you can solve the problem. If you can, say so immediately. However, there may be occasions when you can't do exactly what they would like you to do. In such a situation, try to outline the alternatives or say what you *can* do.

Can you think of any words or phrases you could use to suggest an alternative, instead of simply saying 'No, we can't do that', you could say (jot down your ideas):

-
-

Technique 4: take charge of the situation. Say 'I will' and be positive

To give the client more confidence in you, use: 'I will…' instead of: 'I could…'; 'I might…'; or 'I don't…'; all of which sound weak and negative. For instance, instead of: 'I don't think we can do that. I could try to find out for you'. Say: 'I will go and find out for you.' Using 'will' sounds as if you are really doing something and therefore reassures the client. 'I could try…' sounds vague and leaves the client wondering if anything can or will be done.

Now turn the following statements into ones that begin with '*I will…*'

Rather than:	Try saying:
1. 'Well, I don't know if the Vet is back from lunch yet.'	'*I will…*'
2. 'I don't think we can do anything about that. I could find out for you, I suppose.'	'*I will…*'
3. 'I'm sorry you've had such a bad time. It was not my fault.'	'*I will…*'

Technique 5: tell them what they can do, not what they can't

This is another technique where your response can be positive and active rather than negative and ineffective. Instead of saying 'No', say 'You can…'. This does not always work, as there is not always an alternative. However, there are many situations where you can use this technique. It is much better from the client's point of view to know what they can do rather than what they can't do.

You can use this technique:

- When you cannot give the client exactly what they are asking for, but you have an alternative.
- When you would like to help or show that you want to do so but you are not able to do more than convey your goodwill.
- When your client does not know exactly what he or she wants. Giving customers an option often helps them make their minds up.

Replace each of the following statements with ones beginning with 'You can…'

Instead of:	Try saying:
1. 'I can't help you; I don't know anything about that.'	'You can…'
2. 'You can't get them now and we don't have another one.'	'You can…'
3. 'You can't see him just now; the Practice Manager is not here at the moment.'	'You can…'
4. 'You can't see her today, I'm afraid. She has no more appointments.'	'You can…'

There is one special case that seems to cause the most concern here, and that is when a client asks for the 'umpteenth' repeat prescription. Now, naturally, you will have been told to stick to the rules governing the distribution of animal medicines and tell the client that they can't have a repeat prescription this time (as it has been six months since the vet has seen Moggie) until they have seen the vet. The more you entrench your (correct) position, the more the client will complain that you are being difficult, setting out too much red tape, trying to charge for another consultation… you name it, you've heard it all.

Of course, the worst thing that can happen is for the vet to undermine you by saying (often in full view of the rest of reception) 'Oh that's all right, Mrs Jones, you can have a box of tablets…'

One solution worth a try is to put the responsibility for the pet's welfare back into their hands making sure that they are aware of what they can do:

You: *'Of course you can* have a repeat prescription; *you can* agree with the vet which is the best product, dose, and course of treatment.'

Client: 'I don't want to see the vet; I just want a repeat prescription.'

You: *'I understand you want a repeat prescription and* you can *have one when you've checked with the vet.'*

Client: 'I don't want to see the vet.'

You: *'That's OK. It's your choice. We want to do the best for 'Moggie' and that is best sorted out by the vet'.* You can *see her at 4.30 this afternoon or would tomorrow morning be better for you?* You can *have tonight's dose to tide you over.'*

Client: *'She always lets me have some.'*

You: 'You can *confirm that with her – so would that be this afternoon at 4.30 or tomorrow morning?'*

Client: 'I can't make those times.'

You: 'You can *see her at another time (or of course, another vet) if you wish'.*

SUGGESTED ANSWERS FOR SECTION 4

Technique 2

Ask questions and listen carefully to find out what they want you to do – if anything. Remember that listening to the complaint is sometimes as important as doing something about it.

Technique 3

- 'It is possible to…'
- 'We do have…'
- 'I will check with the Vet when he has finished operating'
- 'I can…but I'm afraid I can't' (putting the positive before the negative).

Technique 4

1. '*I will* see if the manager is available.'
2. '*I will* go and look in the stockroom for you.'
3. '*I will* see that this does not happen again.'

Technique 5

1. '*You can* find out from the manager. I'll go and find her.'
2. '*You can* try an alternative product X. I will find out if we have them in stock.'
3. '*You can* come back tomorrow morning when the practice manager is here. I'll let him know you're coming.' Or 'I can get the practice manager to phone you when he returns.'
4. '*You can* see Mrs Marshall today, or *you can* arrange another appointment with her later in the week…'

SUMMARY

The five techniques outlined in the last section were:

Technique 1:   Solve the problem – rather than blaming yourself or someone else.

Technique 2:   Find out what they want you to do – by asking questions and listening carefully.

Technique 3:   Outline the solution, if there is one, or the alternatives.

Technique 4:   Take charge of the situation. Reassure the client by saying: 'I will…' rather than: 'I could…'; 'You might be able to…'; or 'I don't think…' which sound weak and ineffectual.

Technique 5:   Tell them what they can do, not what they can't do – sound positive and offer an alternative course of action for the client rather than simply saying what they cannot do.

Chapter 9
Fundamentals of first aid

It is hoped that you will never have to refer to this chapter, but occasionally, accidents will happen in the waiting room and you will need to know what to do. The most likely accidents to occur to clients in your waiting room are: fainting, falls, asthma attack, bite wound by dog or cat, and occasionally heart attack.

This chapter is a very basic guide and we recommend that at least one person in the practice attend a First Aid course. In fact, by law, if more than eight people are employed in a workplace a trained First Aider is required. The British Red Cross or St John Ambulance organize courses and a quick look in *Yellow Pages* will provide a telephone contact number.

Do you know where the First Aid box is and who your First Aider is in the practice?

If you find someone lying on the floor the basic rules are as follows, and are easily remembered by DR ABC.

D: Danger   Are you or the casualty in danger?

R: Response   Does your casualty respond to shout/shake or pinch? i.e. conscious or unconscious (Figure 9.1).

A: Airway   Open the airway by gently lifting the chin with two fingers and tilting the head backwards.

B: Breathing   Look, listen and feel for breathing for ten seconds (Figure 9.2).

C: Circulation   Look for movement and check the carotid pulse in the neck for no more than 10 seconds. Check the body for bleeding (Figure 9.3).

If the casualty is unconscious and breathing, you must put them into the recovery position (Figure 9.4).

If the casualty is not breathing, then you should send for help. Get a colleague or someone in the waiting room to phone the ambulance service immediately, remembering to give the following information to the emergency services.

- Full address
- That you have a collapsed male/female, age, not breathing, that you are giving mouth-to-mouth resuscitation.

Figure 9.1   Is the patient conscious? (10 secs)

Figure 9.2   Look, listen, and feel for breathing (10 secs)

Figure 9.3 Check the carotid artery for a pulse (10 secs)

Figure 9.4 For the unconscious and breathing – the recovery position

PROCEDURE FOR NOT BREATHING CASUALTY

Remember every second counts. Lack of oxygen can cause brain damage or death, so do not waste time. It is probably a very good idea for hygienic reasons to have a mouth guard shield in the first aid kit.

- Check mouth and carefully remove any obvious obstruction or false teeth. They may have swallowed their tongue, try to pull it forward.
- Keep the casualty's head tilted back while opening the mouth and pinching the nose firmly.

Figure 9.5   Mouth-to-mouth resuscitation

- Take a full breath and slowly breathe into the mouth until the chest rises, ensure a good seal around the mouth (Figure 9.5).
- Remove your mouth from the casualty and let the chest fall.
- Give a second breath, then look for signs of circulation (see procedure for no circulation below).
- If signs of circulation are present, continue breathing for the casualty.
- If they start to breathe, put them in the recovery position.

NO SIGNS OF CIRCULATION

- Immediately start chest compressions.
- Place heel of hand two fingers width above the junction of the rib margin and breastbone.
- Place other hand on top and interlock your fingers. Keeping arms straight and your fingers off the chest, press down about 4–5 cm.
- Release pressure, keeping your hands in place.
- *Repeat* the compressions 15 times, aiming at a rate of 100 per minute.
- Give 2 more breaths of mouth to mouth.
- Continue 15 compressions to 2 breaths until help arrives.

WHAT TO DO IF A CLIENT FAINTS

Remember the DR ABC: See page 136

1. Remove the pet the client might be holding on to.
2. Check airway, breathing and circulation.
3. Put into recovery position.
4. Keep warm, cover with blankets or coats under as well as over the person.

A CLIENT HAS A HEART ATTACK

A heart attack can occur when one of the blood vessels in the heart becomes blocked. If this happens the heart may stop. Many people who have a heart attack make a good recovery.

You need to be able to recognize the following signs and symptoms:

- Paleness or blueness, around the lips.
- Severe pain in the chest which can spread to the left arm. At onset the client might grasp at their chest because of the pain.
- Sudden faintness or dizziness.
- Breathlessness.
- Sudden collapse.
- Rapid, weak or irregular pulse.

TREATMENT

The conscious casualty

- Place the casualty in the half-seated position, supported behind the back and knees bent, with a folded coat/blanket underneath the knees to give support
- Reassure
- Phone for the ambulance (give details as outlined earlier in this chapter).

Unconscious casualty

- Mouth-to-mouth resuscitation and chest compressions
- Phone for the ambulance (give details as outlined earlier in this chapter).

A CLIENT HAS AN ASTHMA ATTACK

You may recognize when someone is having an attack by:

- Difficulty in breathing
- Wheezing
- Distress
- Anxiety
- Difficulty in speaking
- Blueness of face and lips.

TREATMENT

- Reassure the person.
- Help them to sit down.
- Lean them forward slightly, resting on support.
- Ensure good air supply.
- Give the casualty *their own* medication.
  You will need to call an ambulance if:
- This is the first attack.
- The attack is prolonged and does not respond to medication.
- If the attack appears to be getting worse.

BITE WOUND BY DOG OR CAT

- Remove and restrain the perpetrator, take care, you do not need to be bitten as well.
- Wash and dry your own hands.
- Cover any cuts on your own hands and put on First Aid gloves.
- Clean the cut, if dirty, under running water.
- Pat dry.
- Cover the cut completely with a sterile dressing or plaster.
- If the wound is large or deep it may need suturing, so arrange to get the client to a health centre or hospital accident department.

FOR SEVERE BLEEDING

- Apply direct pressure to the wound using fingers or a pad, yes, even a handkerchief will do and not necessarily recently ironed.
- Raise and support the injured limb, see figure 9.6.
- Lay the casualty down on the floor and treat for shock.
- *Remember!* Protect yourself from infection by wearing gloves; all first aid boxes should have protective gloves. Examination gloves are ideal and ready to hand in the practice. Maybe keep some in a drawer in reception.
- If blood seeps through the bandage *do not* remove it but place a fresh bandage on top, and apply pressure.

FIRST AID BOX

Every practice should have a First Aid box, the Health and Safety (First Aid) Regulations 1981 require employers to provide adequate and appropriate equipment, facilities and personnel to enable first aid to be given if a person is injured or becomes ill at work. It is of course possible to buy ready-filled boxes, however, if you want to make up your own, here are the basic needs, as most practices will have a supply of bandages and dressings to hand. A minimum stock would be:

Figure 9.6   Dealing with severe bleeding from the right forearm

- 20 individually wrapped sterile adhesive dressings (assorted sizes)
- two sterile eye pads
- four individually wrapped triangular bandages (preferably sterile)
- six safety pins
- six medium sized (approx. 12×12 cm) sterile individually wrapped unmedicated wound dressings
- two large (approx. 18×18 cm) sterile individually wrapped unmedicated wound dressings
- one pair of disposable gloves.

You should *not* keep tablets or medicines in the first aid box.

KEEPING RECORDS

By law, it is required that incidents involving injury or illness in the workplace are recorded in an accident book. In these litigious times we live in, and especially when dealing with the public, it is a good idea to record what happened, in case they decide to sue you or your employers.

You can purchase pre-printed Accident books (see further information) or you could make your own, which should record the following information:

- Date, time and place of incident
- Name and job of injured or ill person
- Details of injury/illness and any first aid given
- What happened to the casualty immediately afterwards (for example went to hospital, went home or went back to work)
- Name and signature of person dealing with the incident.

Maybe you should consider taking a first aid course, after all you are likely to be on hand in the reception area if an accident happens. To close on a slightly lighter note, try to avoid placing the client in a recovery kennel, no matter how tempting!

TIPS

- Know location of First Aid box
- Know who is the trained First Aider in the practice.
- Know what to do in an emergency.

FURTHER INFORMATION

Basic Advice on First Aid in the Workplace. Health & Safety Executive
Details of this booklet and other HSE matters can be found on their website.
http:/www.open.gov.uk/home/hsehome.htm
Accident Book. The Stationery Office. Obtainable from any good bookseller
First Aid at Work. Health & Safety Executive.

Chapter 10
Labelling and dispensing

WHAT YOU CAN AND CANNOT DO

NEW REGULATIONS

Dispensing of animal medicines is strictly governed by law and covered in new Veterinary Medicines Regulations 2006 SI 2407, which replaces the 1968 Medicines Act.

Does your practice have a policy on dispensing medicines to clients to meet the new regulations? If not, then it should have.

In legal terms, veterinary medicines are divided into four categories, which you should be conversant with, so that you follow the correct dispensing procedures.

The categories are:

Prescription Only Medicine – Veterinarian (abbreviated to POM-V)
Prescribed by a veterinary surgeon and supplied by either a veterinary surgeon or a pharmacist (*previously POM, MFS and some P products*)

Prescription Only Medicine – Veterinarian, Pharmacist, Suitably Qualified Person (abbreviated to POM-VPS)
Prescribed by any one of the Registered Qualified Persons and supplied by any one of them (*previously PML, MFSX and some P products*)

Non-Food Animal – Veterinarian, Pharmacist, Suitably Qualified Person (abbreviated to NFA-VPS)
Supplied by any one of the Registered Qualified Persons (*previously PML and some P products*)

Authorized Veterinary Medicine – General Sales List (abbreviated to AVM-GSL). Supplied by any retailer (*previously GSL products*)

SQP refers to a Suitably Qualified Person who is registered with a body approved by the Secretary of State, for example a listed Veterinary Nurse who has undertaken Animal Regulations Training Authority (AMTRA) approved training may become an SQP.

Veterinary Surgeons under the 2006 Regulations are listed as Registered Qualified Persons (RQPs) and may retail POM-V, POM-VPS, NFA-VPS, AVM-GSL products.

Now the various categories in more depth.

POM-V

A veterinary medicinal product that has been classified as a POM-V may only be supplied once it has been prescribed by a veterinary surgeon following a clinical assessment of the animal or group of animals. The client may request a written prescription if they do not want the prescribing veterinary surgeon to supply the product. In all cases, the prescribing veterinary surgeon shall accept clinical responsibility for the treatment and the animal or group of animals should be under his/her care.

Any registered veterinary surgeon or registered pharmacist may supply the product against the written prescription. The supplying veterinary surgeon or pharmacist should use their specialist knowledge to check that the prescription accords with their own understanding of the product. If they have concerns about the prescription, they should raise them with the prescribing veterinary surgeon before dispensing the medicine. It is open to any supplier to refuse to supply against a prescription should they wish.

POM-VPS

A veterinary medicinal product classified as POM-VPS may only be prescribed by a Registered Qualified Person (RQP), i.e.:

  i) a registered veterinary surgeon
 ii) a registered pharmacist or
iii) a registered suitably qualified person (SQP).

Again the client may request a written prescription if they do not want the prescribing vet to supply the product. Any vet may supply POM-VPS medicines in accordance with a written prescription from another veterinary surgeon.

A clinical assessment of the animal(s) is not required for this group of veterinary medicines. However, the prescribing vet must, each time they prescribe, be satisfied that the person administering the medicine has the competence to do so safely and that the medicine is intended for its authorized use. The vet must provide advice on how to use the product, taking special account of any warnings or contraindications relevant to the medicine for every prescription. The vet should also take into account directions in Flock/Herd Health Plans, where available, when prescribing.

NFA-VPS

A veterinary medicinal product classified as NFA-VPS may be supplied by a RQP, i.e.:

i) a registered veterinary surgeon
ii) a registered pharmacist or
iii) a registered suitably qualified person (SQP).

Clinical assessments are not required for supply of this category of medicine.

As with POM-VPS, the vet must be satisfied that the person buying the medicine is competent to use it and will be aware of conditions of use.

A product will generally be included in the NFA-VPS category when:

- it is indicated for use only in non-food animals
- it is used routinely to prevent or limit the effects of endemic disease in non-food animals
- its use implies risks for the user, the animal, for consumer safety or for the environment, but users can be made aware of suitable countermeasures through simple, oral or written, advice
- the animal keeper can be given sufficient practical advice to permit effective/safe usage.

AVM–GSL

A veterinary medicinal product classified as an AVM-GSL may be supplied by any retailer, i.e. saddlers or animal health merchants.

A product will generally be included in the AVM-GSL category when:

- its use has a wide margin of safety
- it is used to alleviate or prevent the symptoms of disease or support the treatment of common ailments
- special advice is not required to permit safe/effective use.

Supply when a veterinary surgeon is not present

The veterinary surgeon need not be present when the product is handed over but, if not present, he/she must:

- authorize each transaction before the product is handed over
- be satisfied that the person who hands it over is competent to do so.

In the age of the Internet pharmacy, a client may legally request a prescription for a product.

A prescription may be verbal or in writing. Prescribing is considered to be the action of deciding, instructing and recording which treatment should be administered to an animal. It can be carried out by any registered qualified person (RQP), i.e. a veterinary surgeon, pharmacist or suitably qualified person, according to the distribution category of the veterinary medicinal product concerned. Generally, most written prescriptions are expected to be provided by veterinary surgeons. A written prescription is required when the product is to be supplied by a person working at a different business or site from where the product was prescribed by another RQP. The sites may be within or outside the same authorized premises, but the important point is that they are geographically separate. The animal owner should then give the written prescription to the person supplying the product. As the prescribing RQP will have completed the required records held at that site, a written prescription is not necessary when the prescribing and supplying RQPs are working on the same site.

As well as specifying an authorized veterinary medicinal product, a prescription from a veterinary surgeon may be for a product that has been prescribed under the cascade. In these cases, the prescription may be written for a human medicine or a preparation that is to be made up to meet the particular circumstances. Veterinary surgeons must note on prescriptions for human medicines that the product has been prescribed under the cascade and it is helpful for the supplier if this is done for all cascade prescriptions.

PRESCRIPTIONS

There is no particular format for a written veterinary prescription, but prescribers must include the following information:

- Name, address and telephone number of the person prescribing the product
- Qualifications of the person providing the prescription, MRCVS or the SQP registration number
- Name and address of the owner or keeper
- Premises at which the animals are kept if this is different from the address of the owner or keeper
- Species of animal, identification and number of the animals
- Date of the prescription
- Signature or other authentication of the person prescribing the product
- Name and amount of the product prescribed
- Dosage and administration instructions
- Any necessary warnings
- Withdrawal period.

Practices must take reasonable steps to ensure that a prescription is genuine and prescribers may choose to use various methods, such as stickers or serial numbers, to help with this. If there is any doubt about the validity of a prescription, then a telephone conversation with the prescriber should be regarded as a minimum step to confirm its validity.

UNCERTAINTY

If you are in any doubt as to whether or not you can supply, or what to supply, check with a vet before you do. Ultimately, it is a veterinary responsibility, and you must allow the decision to be made by the vet.

DRUG ENQUIRIES

Drug enquiries may be about their supply, their availability, their price, their uses and efficacy or their restrictions.

SUPPLY

General advice

In general, you should remember that the practice is allowed to supply the few products that are on the general sale list (AVM-GSL), such as fly repellent for horses, to anyone who asks for them. The same goes for non-drug supplies such as marking sprays, or lamb teats. It is only allowed to supply products on the pharmacy and merchants' list NFA-VPS or POM-V to its own clients, for use in their animals that are under the care of one or more of the practice's vets.

If the enquiring customer is not a client, you will need to explain this law to them politely. If they are not immediately satisfied with this answer, you should ask a vet or the SQP to speak to them.

POLICY

Your employers will have their own policy as to how they interpret the law with regard to supplying drugs. You must make yourself familiar with their intentions, and stick to them. If there isn't a detailed set of standing instructions, you should ask for one. It may be your responsibility to help in implementing the policy, but it is not your responsibility to design it.

CHECKING

Always check the species for which medicine is required, the number of animals, the age and sex and, for many medicines, the weight. These as well as the name and address of the owner are vital details to know before you can take any further action.

RECORDS

RECORD KEEPING

It is the responsibility of the SQP who prescribes a POM–VPS product to keep the documents relating to the prescription or make a record of it, irrespective of who supplies it. The following must be recorded in each case:

- name and address of the recipient
- identity of the product including its name, strength and pharmaceutical form
- quantity
- date
- if it is against a written prescription, who provided the prescription
- batch number
- the expiry date.

It is good practice for an SQP who supplies an NFA-VPS product and carries out the related SQP duties in respect of the supply, to keep the related documents or make a record of the information as set out above.

It is not necessary to keep individual records which tie receipt of a batch of product to its individual supply providing it is possible, using all the records together, to identify which batch has been supplied to which person and carry out a full batch recall if necessary.

RECORD KEEPING OF PURCHASES

When a drug order is received from the wholesaler, often the receptionist is responsible for helping to check the order in. They should be aware of what must be recorded regarding receipt of POM-VPS products or make a record of at least the following:

- identity of the product including its name, strength and pharmaceutical form
- date of receipt
- name and address of the supplier
- quantity
- batch number
- expiry date.

The documents or record must be kept for at least 5 years. It is good practice to keep these records in respect of all authorized veterinary medicinal products.

Practices will be expected to carry out a detailed audit at least once a year of all the transactions, with incoming and outgoing products being reconciled with products held in stock. These records will be kept for a period of 3 years, and may be inspected by Veterinary Surgeons from Animal Health (formerly the State Veterinary Services). Also the Veterinary Medicines Directorate has a team of inspectors. Penalties for failing to keep the necessary records could, on conviction, result in either a fine or imprisonment, or both.

Naturally, recording the supply will be important because it needs invoicing to the client, or a cash receipt. There may be other records to be kept as well (see current legislation). Some stock control systems require a supply to be noted so that it can be deducted from the stock report. Some marketing policies on behalf of pharmaceutical companies will require the recording and monitoring of the sale of particular lines.

REPEAT PRESCRIPTIONS

Some practices have different policies to deal with large and small animal repeat requests. It is always sensible to allow only a certain amount of time to elapse before the animal must be examined again by a vet to allow further prescriptions. This is always more difficult to implement in farm animals, rather than in horses or small animals. Whatever the policies are, you must find out and stick to them, except when authorized to make an exception by a vet. You must not make judgements on your own initiative.

PROBLEMS

If you have problems explaining the practice's own rules, or the law, to a client, always say that you will check with a vet as soon as possible. Do so while the client is still on the premises, if possible. The vet can then make a decision and explain it to the client. Remember, if you are making contact with a vet by mobile phone, always let them know that the client can hear what is being said, before they start to speak. 'I have got Mr Spencer with me, he is asking if he can have some more penicillin for his calves.' The reason for letting the vet know that the client is there is to avoid them saying something about the client they might regret!

AVAILABILITY

Is it stocked?

If you are asked whether you stock a particular product, always answer straightforwardly. If you don't stock it, leave it there. Find out what it is required for, suggest that you might have alternatives, or if you haven't any, that you might be able to stock the product from now on, and offer to reply later. Check with a vet, and make sure the response is made.

Is it in stock?

If you are asked whether you have stocks of a product that you normally do stock, find out how much is needed, check the situation and reply honestly. If you have to answer 'no', or that you haven't enough, never leave it there. Always explain when your next supply will be. If you are in any doubt, offer to contact your supplier and find out. If you have promised to do so, make sure you do. It is a good policy to phone the client when the stock comes in rather than asking them to call back in a few days time, when you expect to have stock. Most wholesalers offer a next day delivery service.

PRICE

Enquiries about price and discounts

What is the practice policy regarding handling enquiries? Are you allowed to quote prices without first referring to either the practice manager or vet? Price of medicines is a somewhat emotive subject, especially with farm clients. If you don't have any guidelines from your employer, ask for some.

USES AND EFFICACY

Non-specific

Some enquiries are of a very general nature, such as: 'Have you got something I could use for...?' Unless the answers fall into the category NFA-GSL, bearing in mind the practice policy, you should always take veterinary advice before responding to the request.

Some enquiries are only slightly more specific, such as 'Could I have some "white drench" for lambs?' Again, the practice policy will dictate what your response should be.

Even if you are allowed to dispense it (only if you are an SQP), you must be very sure what the client means and, if you are in any doubt, take advice. The best advice would be to check with a vet in any case.

Specific

Requests for advice such as, 'Will these mastitis tubes treat streptococcal mastitis?' or 'Can I use the Vetiocillin I had for the calves, on my lambs?' should always be redirected to a vet. Do not take the responsibility of answering, even if you overheard the same request and the answer to it yesterday. You may very well feel able to answer, 'Does the Dogovac Parvo-CXX booster my dog had last week only cover parvovirus?', but unless you are equipped to ask what other vaccinations it has had in the past and advise on their effect as well, always make it plain you are answering that specific question alone. Otherwise, and if you are in any doubt as to why the question has been asked, redirect to the vet.

RESTRICTION

Withdrawal times

Practice policy will dictate whether or not you are empowered to answer queries about the withdrawal times of drugs. If you are, don't rely on your memory, and always make sure you are using the most up-to-date reference book. The NOAH Compendium of Data Sheets is hardly ever good enough, as information can be dated by the time it is in print. The most recent Withdrawal Periods List, also published by NOAH, is likely to be the best source of information. A quick check of the NOAH website, www.noahcompendium.co.uk, will give you the information needed. Remember the statutory withdrawal period rules and that there are differences between species. Even if you have the authority to advise, don't hesitate to check your advice with a vet or an SQP. If you don't have the authority, redirect your enquiry to the vet or the SQP in the practice.

If you have had to redirect any enquiry to a vet or SQP whom you are unable to contact immediately for a reply, *always* make sure the request has been answered by checking with the person concerned.

LABELLING

Part of the business of labelling medicaments is covered by the law, Veterinary Medicines Regulations 2006 and by the RCVS codes of practice, and your vets have the responsibility of complying with them. That ought to make it your responsibility as well. So be aware of what is contained in these two pieces of legislation.

Every medicament that goes out of the surgery must carry a label giving very well defined information. It must be indelible and legible. That means that mechanically printed labels are probably best, and some practices, like most pharmacies, use computer printers already. But failing this, biro, roller ball or felt tip pens are acceptable, but fountain pen and pencil are not, as they can be erased.

The essential information that the product should be labelled with is:

1. The name and address of the owner of the animal.
2. The identity of the animal it is intended for.
3. The name and address of the veterinary surgeon.
4. The date of dispensing.
5. The words 'For animal treatment only'.
6. The words 'For external use only', if applicable.
7. The words 'Keep out of reach of children' or with the same meaning.
8. The withdrawal periods, if the medication is for food animals. Remember, horses are regarded as food animals under EU legislation.

In addition to this, it is recommended that the following information is included also:

1. The name, size, strength of the product.
2. Directions of use.
3. Any warnings related to the use of the product.

Some of this is often already printed on the product's label by the manufacturer. If so, it is important that none of it is obscured by the practice's own label. Often this is very difficult to achieve, so the label for Sesoral tablets might read:

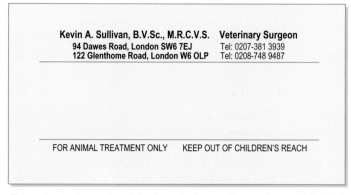

Kevin A. Sullivan, B.V.Sc., M.R.C.V.S.   Veterinary Surgeon
94 Dawes Road, London SW6 7EJ   Tel: 0207-381 3939
122 Glenthome Road, London W6 OLP   Tel: 0208-748 9487

FOR ANIMAL TREATMENT ONLY   KEEP OUT OF CHILDREN'S REACH

Figure 10.1   Example of the layout of a small animal practice's label

For animal treatment only
Animal: Moggie
Owner: Ms J Hoggetal, Cobwebs, Elder Street,
Wimbish, Saffron Walden
24/8/08
Directions: day 1: 4 tablets by mouth morning and evening
days 2–5: 3 tablets morning and evening
Keep out of the reach and sight of children
Anywhere Veterinary Group
4 Castle Walk, Saffron Walden, Essex

and for the Ventocillin Injection, in its original bottle:

For animal treatment only
Owner: J Durrani, The Byre, Hants
10/10/08
Directions: give 15 ml daily by intramuscular injection, for 3 days
Withdrawal periods: milk – 24 hours meat – 21 days
Keep out of reach and sight of children
Spring Veterinary Group
4 Castle Parade, Newtown, Hants

and for PEP powder, in its original pack:

For animal treatment only
Animal: calves
Owner: G Smith, Waytown
6-8–08
Directions: apply directly to both eyes twice daily
For external use only
Keep out of reach and sight of children
Bridgetown Veterinary Group
4 Castle Parade, Bridgetown, Staffs

CONTAINERS FOR TABLETS

It is not acceptable any longer for the only container of medicinal products to be a paper envelope or plastic bag.

If the tablets are in a manufacturer's blister pack, or strip, then the outer container can be a paper or cardboard carton or wallet. It is not always easy to make these look very professional, and it may be worth a look around to see what is available to improve the presentation of blister packs, while allowing a clear

VALLEY VETERINARY GROUP

TUTTS CLUMP, BRADFIELD, BERKSHIRE.   Tel: (01734) 744352

NAME	ANIMAL
ADDRESS	DOSE
	WITHDRAWAL PERIOD
	MEAT MILK
DATE	

KEEP OUT OF REACH OF CHILDREN   FOR ANIMAL TREATMENT ONLY

Figure 10.2   Example of a Farm Animal practice label. (Grateful thanks to Malling Press for supplying examples of labels)

label to be added. Loose tablets are best dispensed in child-resistant containers, but some old people have difficulty with these, and perhaps should be given the option of a different lid. A sign in the waiting room should inform clients that there is an option.

Naturally, this is not appropriate for tablets or pessaries for farm animals, but the need to label these products still applies, and some form of container is often necessary.

Quite apart from the legal requirements of labelling and containers, do remember that everything that comes out of the surgery is sending messages to your clients. If it is seen by non-clients, it will be sending messages to them as well. So it is important that the messages are the right ones, the ones you want to convey. Messages about:

1. efficiency
2. care
3. cleanliness
4. professionalism.

Even if it is only a clear presentation of the practice name and telephone number, you ought to make sure that no opportunity is lost in marketing the benefits of the practice in this way. Don't just slap a label on at any angle, line it up with the design of the pack. That way your practice is part of the overall visual appeal of the pack, not a distraction.

It is important to retain as much of the manufacturer's efforts at presentation as possible. A damaged box or a scruffy container reduces the value of what is inside. Of course, it doesn't really make any difference to how the drug works, or how many animals it will treat, but it reduces the perception of the value to the client who has purchased it. He or she won't be wondering whether it is any good or not, but it may just occur to him that he's paying too much for it.

If goods arrive damaged from the wholesaler, they should be sent back, and it follows that you need to look after the packaging of your own stock on the shelf, too. That may mean not overstocking, it may mean not piling it too high, it may mean choosing a brand that packs well on a shelf, rather than one that packs badly, if there is a choice.

GENERAL CHECKLIST WHEN DEALING WITH VARIOUS ASPECTS OF DISPENSING

- Is the owner a client?
- When was the animal last seen in the case of a repeat prescription?
- Who was the veterinary surgeon who authorized the sale?
- State of container or package professional in the case of returned product?
- Have you completed the record card?
- In the case of a query did the product come from your practice?

FURTHER READING AND INFORMATION

The Royal College of Veterinary Surgeons, London *RCVS Guide to Professional Conduct*.
   Tel:+44(0)207 222 2001 Fax: +44(0)207 222 2004 www.rcvs.org.uk

British Veterinary Association, London *Code of Practice on Medicines*.
   Tel:+44 (0) 207636 6541
   Fax: +44 (0) 207908 6349 www.bva.co.uk

Veterinary Medicines Directorate, Weybridge, Surrey
   Phone : +44 (0)1932 338319 Fax: +44 (0)1932 336618 www.vmd.gov.uk

National Office of Animal Health (NOAH) Enfield, Middlesex
   Phone: +44 (0)20 8367 3131
   Fax +44 (0)20 8363 1155
   www.noah.com and www.noahcompendium.co.uk

AMTRA (Animal Medicines Training Regulatory Authority) Woodbridge Suffolk
   Tel: +44 (0)1394 411010
   Fax: +44 (0)1394 410455
   Email: info@amtra.org.uk

Action plan – copy this blank outline for future use

I will do this:	With this support:	With this outcome:	By this date:
e.g. Check that I am always welcoming on the phone	*Talk to my colleagues about it*	*Measure how clients respond through a waiting room questionnaire (see page 41)*	*Review again in three months time*

Index

A

Acceptance, body language, 39
Accessibility, 8
Accident book, 142–3
Accidents, 136–43
Aggressive behaviour, 93–7
    refusals, 113–15
    in response to complaints, 106–7
        consequences of, 109
Angry clients, 102, 117
Apologizing, 103–4, 124
Appointment making, 10–13
Assertiveness, 93–7, 105–13
    ABC response pattern, 106–7
    in action, 110–13
    communication, 111–12
    core statements, 112–13
    quiz, 94–6
    responding to complaints, 105–13
    rewards of, 110
    saying no, 113–15
    style, self-test, 107–8
    training, 78
Assuming, listening, 34
Asthma attacks, 140–1
Attitude, 29
Augmented product, 14, 17–18
Authorized Veterinary Medicine - General
    Sales List (AVM-GSL), 144, 146–7
Awkward situations, stress and, 90–1

B

Barriers to excellence, 18–19
'Be perfect' stress driver, 82–3
'Be strong' stress driver, 85–6
Bites, dog or cat, 141
Bleeding, severe, 141
Body language, 38–41
Breathing, casualty not, 138–9
'Broken record' no, 114–15

C

Call monitoring systems, 61
Casualties
    no signs of circulation, 139
    not breathing, 138–9
Chest compression, 139
'Chuffed Chart,' 1, 2
Circulation, no signs of, 139
Client care equation, 4, 6
Client(s)
    definition of, 4
    difficult *see* Difficult clients
    feedback *see* Feedback, client
    focusing on *see* Focus, client
    making feel special *see* Special, making
        clients feel
    needs *see* Needs, client
    service *see* Client service
    uniqueness, 42
    valuing, 19
Client service, 1–25
    barriers to excellence, 18–19
    client assessment of, 16–19
    defined, 5
    making clients feel special *see* Special,
        making clients feel
    monitoring, 24
    planning for excellence, 19
    plan of action, 20–4
    quality
        client definition of, 8–9
        general definition of, 5–6
        of health care, 24
        influence on consumers, 13–15
        meaning of, 6–8
    solutions, 119–35
    'step-by-step' in practice, 9–13
    valuing the client, 19
    why bother?, 1–4
Closed questions, 36–7
Comments, 98 *see also* Complaints; Feedback,
    client

Communication
    assertive, 111–12
    client focus, 32–3
    clients perception of, 8
    non-verbal, 38–41
    objectives, 32–3
    skills, stress reduction, 78
    special needs clients, 54, 55–6
Competence, 8
Complaints, 98–118
    apologizing, 103–4
    assertiveness, 105–13
    being genuine, 104–5
    cooperation techniques, 132–5
    dos and don'ts, 116–17
    general guidelines for handling, 102–5
    generating solutions, 130–5
    handling specific types of people, 117–18
    key tips, 116–18
    listening to the client, 102–3, 104
    positive thinking, 99–101
    procedure, 130–1
    quiz, 100–1
    reasons for, 119–21
    saying no, 113–15
    ten-point plan, 105–6, 116
    thinking like a client, 102
    turning into opportunities, 101
    your rights, 115–16
Compliments, 98
Concentrating, listening, 34
Confidence, body language, 39
Confidentiality of fax messages, 66
Cooperation, body language, 39
Core statements, 112–13
Courtesy, 8
Credibility, 8
    body language, 39
Criticizing, mentally, 35

D

Daydreaming, 35
Defensiveness, body language, 38
Difficult clients
    dealing with, 125–7
    stress and, 90–1
Difficult situations, 90–2
Difficult telephone calls, 63–4
Dispensing *see* Labelling and dispensing
Doubt, body language, 38
DR ABC mnemonic, 136
Dress, 29–30
Drivers and stress, 82–7

Drug(s)
    containers, 153–5
    enquiries, 147–8, 150–1
    withdrawal times, 151 *see also* Labelling
        and dispensing

E

Empathy, 50, 124
Empowerment, staff, 23
Enhanced product, 13–14
Evaluation, body language, 38
Excellence
    barriers to, 18–19
    planning for, 19
Exercise and stress, 78
Expectations, client, 3, 5
Expression, 50
Eye contact, 26

F

Facilities, 16–17
Fainting, 140
Fax messages, 65–6
Feedback, client, 23
First aid, 136–43
First Aid box, 141–2
First impressions, 26–31
    before answering the phone, 30–1
    first few seconds, 26–7
    lasting impressions, 31
    moments of truth, 27–8
    waiting room, 28–9
Focus, client, 32–41
    face-to-face, 32–3
    giving 110%, 41
    listening, 33–6
    non-verbal communication, 38–41
    questioning, 36–8

G

Generic product, 13, 17
Goal setting, 22

H

Handling information, 127–30
Head receptionist(s)
    commitment to client service, 20
    pressure, 70–1

Health care quality, 24
Healthy eating, 78
Hearing impaired clients, 52–4
Heart attacks, 140
Honesty
    body language, 39
    building trust, 48–9
'Hurry up' stress driver, 84–5

I

Information handling, 127–30
Intangibles, building, 17–18

J

Judging, mentally, 35

K

Know-it-all clients, handling, 117–18
Knowledge and quality, 8

L

Labelling and dispensing, 144–55
    checklist, 155
    drug enquiries, 147–8, 150–1
    labels, 151–3
    new regulations
        AVM-GSL, 144, 146–7
        NFA-VPS, 144, 145–6
        POM-V, 144, 145
        POM-VPS, 144, 145
    prescriptions, 147
        repeat, 149
    record keeping, 148–55
    tablet containers, 153–5
Leading questions, 37
Liability, 8
Listening, 33–6, 50
    assuming, 34
    to clients problems, 122
    to complaints, 102–3, 104
    concentrating, 34
    daydreaming, 35
    finishing sentences, 35
    mentally judging and/or criticizing, 35
    quiz, 51
    skills, 36

Listening (*Continued*)
    status, 35
    summary of effective, 35–6
    switching off, 34
    on the telephone, 68
    thinking ahead, 34

M

Managers, pressure, 70–1
Moments of truth, 27–8
Monitoring, service, 24
MORI poll, 1–2
Motivation, staff, 22–3

N

Needs, client, 5, 52–7
    identifying, 21
    putting first, 22
    special, 52–7
Negative body language, 40
Negative comments *see* Complaints
Nervousness, body language, 39
NFA-VPS, 144, 145–6
NLP (neuro-linguistic programming), 87–9,
    99–101
No, saying, 113–15
NOAH, 151
Non-Food Animal - Veterinarian, Pharmacist,
    Suitably Qualified Person (NFA-VPS),
    144, 145–6
Non-verbal communication, 38–41
Notice board, 28

O

Openness, body language, 38
Open questions, 37

P

Passive behaviour, 93–7
    in response to complaints, 107
        consequences of, 109–10
Perception, client, 5, 6, 19
Performance measures, 22
Personality, professional, 44–5
Phone skills *see* Telephone skills
'Please' stress driver, 83–4

PLUS acronym, 42
POM-V, 144, 145
POM-VPS, 144, 145
Positive body language, 40
Positive thinking, 99–101 *see also* NLP
    (neuro-linguistic programming)
Posters, promotional, 28
Potential offering, 14, 18
Prescription Only Medicine – Veterinarian,
    Pharmacist, Suitably Qualified Person
    (POM-VPS), 144, 145
Prescription Only Medicine – Veterinarian
    (POM-V), 144, 145
Prescriptions, 147
    repeat, 149
Pressure, 70–97 *see also* Stress
Price
    customer perception of, 16
    influence on consumers, 13
    quality and, 16
Problems, clients
    acknowledging, 122–3, 124
    case study, 123
    cooperation techniques, 132–5
    difficult clients *see* Difficult clients
    generating solutions, 130–5
    handling information, 127–30
    owning, 122–3, 124–5
    reasons for, 119–21
    understanding, 121–3 *see also* Complaints
Product purchase, deciding factors in,
    13–14
Product quality, influence on consumers,
    13–14
Professional personality, 44–5
Promotions, 17
Puzzlement, body language, 38

Q

Qualitative information, 128
Quality
    client definition of, 8–9
    health care, 24
    meaning of, 6–8
Quantitative information, 128
Questioning, 36–8
    checklist, 38
    clients problems, 122
    closed questions, 36–7
    leading questions, 37
    open questions, 37
Queue management, 92–3
Quo vadis study, 2–3

R

Rapport, building, 45–7
Reassurance, body language, 39
Recognition, staff, 23
Record keeping
    accidents, 142–3
    labelling and dispensing, 148–55
Recovery position, 136, 137–8
Refusing requests, 113–15
Registered Qualified Person (RQP), 144,
    145, 146
Rejection, body language, 38
Relationships
    developing, 45–7
    quiz, 46–7
Repeat prescriptions, 149
Respect, 49
Responsiveness, 8
Rewards, staff, 23
Rights, human, 115–16
Rude clients, handling, 117

S

Satisfaction, client, 5
    client definition of, 8–9
Security, 8
Self-control, body language, 39
Self-talk, 87–9
Sensitivity, 50
Service *see* Client service
Sincerity, body language, 39
Smiling, 26–7
    over the phone, 62
    responding to forced, 44
Solutions, generating, 130–5
Special, making clients feel, 42–57
    checklist, 57
    clients needs, 52–7
    developing relationships and building
        rapport, 45–7
    golden rules, 42–4, 47–52
    key tips, 57
    professional personality, 44–5
    uniqueness, 42
Special needs clients, 52–7
Speech impaired clients, 55–7
Staff
    empowerment, 23
    motivation, 22–3
    recognition, 23
    rewards, 23
    training, 23, 60

Strengths, practice, 21
Stress, 70–97
  advanced management, 78–87
  checklist, 72
  levels of, 71–4
  minimizing, 76–87
    long-term resilience, 77–8
    short-term measures, 76–7
  reaction types, 75–6
  removing from difficult situations, 90–3
  risk assessment, 73–4
  self-talk/NLP, 87–9
  symptoms of, 74–6
  time off work, 70
  tips for remaining professional, 97
Suitably Qualified Person (SQP), 144, 145
Suspicion, body language, 38
Suspicious clients, handling, 117
Switching off, 34
Sympathy, 50, 124

T

Tablet containers, 153–5
Telephone skills, 58–69
  before answering, 30–1
  automated handling systems, 61
  checklist, 69
  difficult calls, 63–4
  don't list, 66–7
  fax messages, 65–6
  making calls, 62–5
  practice phone policy, 59–62
  preparation for incoming calls, 59
  preparation for making calls, 62–3
  proactive phone use, 67–9

Telephone skills (*Continued*)
  problems, 64–5
  seven P's, 67
  unwanted calls, 65
Thinking ahead, listening, 34
Time management, 78
Training, staff
  answering the phone, 60
  in general, 23
Transactional Analysis, 78–87
Trust, building, 48–52
  quiz, 51
'Try hard' stress driver, 86–7

U

Understanding, 50

V

Values, 50
Valuing the client, 19
Visually impaired clients, 54–5

W

Waiting room first impressions, 28–9
Waiting times, 16
Wants, client, 5
Weaknesses, practice, 21
Whingeing clients, handling, 117
Withdrawal times, drug, 151
Work/life balance, 78
Wounds, first aid, 141